100 Epic Mediterranean Recipes

The Ultimate Cookbook of 100+ Recipes to Reset Your Metabolism and Change your Eating Habits

Table of Contents

INTRODUCTION 7

CHAPTER 1. RICE AND GRAINS 10

1. Long-Grain Rice Congee and Vietnamese Chicken 10
2. Wild Rice Soup and Creamy Chicken 11
3. Best Spanish rice 12
4. Classic Rice Pilaf 13
5. Sarah's Rice Pilaf 14
6. Homemade Fried Rice 15
7. Cranberry Rice 16
8. Kickin' Rice 17
9. Garlic Rice 18
10. Sweet Rice 19
11. Gourmet Mushroom Risotto 20
12. John's Beans and Rice 21
13. Creamy Chicken and Wild Rice Soup 23
14. Carrot Rice 24
15. Rice Sauce 24
16. Brown Rice 25
17. Rice Lasagna 26
18. Rice Milk 27
19. Breakfast Salad from Grains and Fruits 28
20. Puttanesca Style Bucatini 29

21.	Sausage and Bean Casserole	30
22.	Hot Vegetarian Two-Bean Cassoulet	31
23.	Moroccan Spiced Couscous	32
24.	Bulgur Tabbouleh	33
25.	Parmesan and Collard Green Oats	34
26.	Italian Barley with Artichoke Hearts	35
27.	Vegetable Rice Bowl	36
28.	Cherry Tomato Rice Pilaf with Pistachios	37
29.	Italian Cannellini Beans with Egg Noodles	38
30.	Spicy Garbanzo Bowl with Feta Cheese	39
31.	Chickpea and Rice	41
32.	One-Pot Rice and Chicken	42
33.	Grain Bowl with Lentil and Chickpeas	43
34.	White Beans with Vegetables	45
35.	Yangchow Chinese Style Fried Rice	46
36.	Seafood and Veggie Pasta	47
37.	Seafood Paella with Couscous	48
38.	Shrimp Paella Made with Quinoa	50
39.	Shrimp, Lemon and Basil Pasta	51
40.	Simple Penne Anti-Pasto	52
41.	Spaghetti in Lemon Avocado White Sauce	53
42.	Spanish Rice Casserole with Cheesy Beef	54
43.	Squash and Eggplant Casserole	56

44.	Stuffed Tomatoes with Green Chili	57
45.	Tasty Lasagna Rolls	59
46.	Tasty Mushroom Bolognese	61
47.	Tortellini Salad with Broccoli	62
48.	Turkey and Quinoa Stuffed Peppers	63
49.	Veggie Pasta with Shrimp, Basil and Lemon	64
50.	Veggies and Sun-Dried Tomato Alfredo	65

CHAPTER 2. DESSERTS 67

1.	Dessert Pie	67
2.	Date Balls	68
3.	Sugar-coated Pecans	68
4.	Jalapeño Popper Spread	69
5.	Delicious French Eclairs	70
6.	Sweet Tropical Medley Smoothie	71
7.	Ginger Pineapple	72
8.	Roasted Berry and Honey Yogurt Pops	72
9.	Key Lime Pie	73
10.	Healthy Zucchini Pudding	74
11.	Chocolate Ganache	75
12.	Simple Peanut Butter and Chocolate Balls	76
13.	Mango Bowls	77
14.	Walnut Apple Pear Mix	77
15.	Spiced Pear Sauce	78

16.	Blueberry Yogurt Mousse	79
17.	Stuffed Plums	80
18.	Cocoa Sweet Cherry Cream	80
19.	Mango and Honey Cream	81
20.	Cinnamon Pears	82
21.	Classic Fig Clafoutis	83
22.	Semolina Cake with Almonds	84
23.	Romantic Mug Cakes	85
24.	Pistachio and Tahini Halva	86
25.	Authentic Greek Rizogalo	87
26.	Greek Frozen Yogurt Dessert	88
27.	Salted Pistachio and Tahini Truffles	89
28.	Traditional Olive Oil Cake with Figs	90

CHAPTER 3. SNACKS 92

29.	Jazzed-Up Olives	92
30.	Olive Tapenade	93
31.	Spicy Chickpeas	93
32.	Layered Hummus Dip	94
33.	Kibbeh (Lebanese Croquettes)	95
34.	Cheese Plate with Fruit and Crackers	97
35.	Radicchio Stuffed With Goat Cheese and Salmon	98
36.	Rosemary–Sea Salt Crackers with Lemon-Parsley Dip	99
37.	Spinach and Artichoke Dip	101

38. Stuffed Cherry Tomatoes 102
39. Spiced Baked Pita Chips 102
40. Roasted Red Pepper Dip 103
41. Deviled Eggs with Spanish Smoked Paprika 104
42. Aperol Spritz 105
43. VIN Brule 106
44. Plum Wraps 107
45. Easy Medi Kale 108
46. Tropical Pineapple Smoothie 108
47. Radish Bowls 109
48. Cheddar Bites 110
49. Creamy Pepper Spread 111

Introduction

The Mediterranean diet doesn't explicitly exclude any food group; it simply promotes better food choices such as replacing bad fats with good fats, red meat with seafood, and so on. It promotes foods that are as close to their natural state as possible. The Mediterranean diet is one of the easiest diets to follow, as well as one of the best diets for a wide range of chronic diseases. It has been shown to lower the risk of diabetes, cardiovascular disease, and cancer. The Mediterranean diet may help you lose unwanted pounds and slow the aging process by five to ten years. But what makes the eating habits of the Italians and Greeks such a genius diet plan is that it's not just about food; it's a whole lifestyle! Over the decades, the Mediterranean diet saw a slow rise in the Western world. Many countries of the west were slow to pick it up, but once they did, they realized that they had discovered the key to the Elixir of Life. The Mediterranean diet not only helped people rely on a wholesome and healthy diet, but it helped them lose weight, power up their immune systems, improved their vitality, and even contributed to healthy skin. In other words, the Mediterranean diet helped people feel good and look good. The combination of benefits changed people's perception of what they should be having and question their eating habits.

For example, many people often skip breakfast because they feel that having a meal in the morning adds more weight to their bodies. However, the Mediterranean diet does not skip breakfast. On the contrary, it considers breakfasting the most important meal of the day. The countries that relied on the Mediterranean diet saw their benefits way before any scientific research was conducted. They didn't have any research conducted to guide them toward a particular eating pattern or food content. Essentially, the diet has been refined over millennia, as newer methods of cooking were introduced. But the adherence to a healthy form of the diet remained, no matter how old the diet grew.

It all comes down to what we eat when we eat it, and in what quantities. The Mediterranean diet is the traditional diet of the people of the Mediterranean area. It has been shown to be healthier than typical American and British diets. This diet contains plenty of fresh fruits, vegetables, and fish. It also allows for whole grains instead of refined white rice like other diets. The Mediterranean diet is considered a low glycemic dietary pattern, meaning it will not spike your blood sugar levels. It contains many vitamins and minerals that help to support a healthy heart and a strong immune system.

This book has been written specifically for people who want to get into this healthy way of eating. It will teach you how the Mediterranean diet can change your life forever!

For centuries, people have been cutting back on unhealthy foods and adding more healthy foods to their diet. Yet, for some reason, this good habit seems to have stopped before it even started. Not anymore. In "Mediterranean Diet Meal Preparation", you'll learn the secrets to losing belly Fat: and getting your body into better shape.

This book will show you how you can:

Get healthy with new food choices. Get more energy.

Lose belly Fat: without dieting; take advantage of homemade meal-preparation methods. Find healthy alternatives for traditional treats. Get the right nutrients.

The Mediterranean could be considered as a decorative and beautiful plant.

In the Mediterranean region, there are so many palm trees that give the area a resort feel. However, the plant has gained popularity in recent years because it has various health benefits. This diet emphasizes foods that are fresh, whole, unprocessed, and minimally altered. Benefits of eating the Mediterranean way include a lower risk of heart disease, cancer, stroke, depression, obesity, and diabetes.

Chapter 1. Rice and Grains

1. Long-Grain Rice Congee and Vietnamese Chicken

Preparation Time: 10 minutes
Cooking Time: 18 minutes
Servings: 4
Ingredients:

- 1/8 cup uncooked jasmine rice
- 1 whole chicken
- 3 pieces fresh ginger root
- 1 stalk of lemongrass
- 1 tablespoon salt
- 1/4 cup chopped coriander
- 1/8 cup chopped fresh chives
- Ground black pepper to taste
- 1 lime, cut into 8 quarters

Directions:

1. Place the chicken in a pan. Pour enough water to cover the chicken. Merge the ginger, lemongrass, and salt; bring to a boil. Lower the heat, cover, and let it simmer for 1 hour to an hour and a half.
2. Filter the broth and put the broth back in a pan. Allow the chicken to cool, then remove the bones and skin and tear them into small pieces; put aside.
3. Attach the rice to the broth and bring to a boil. Turn the heat to medium and cook for 30 minutes, stirring occasionally. Adjust if necessary with extra water or salt. The congee is done, but you can still cook for 45 minutes for better consistency.

4. Pour the congee into bowls and garnish with chicken, coriander, chives, and pepper. Squeeze the lime juice to taste.

Nutrition:

- Calories: 642
- Fat: 42.3 g
- Carbohydrates: 9.8 g
- Protein: 53 g

2. Wild Rice Soup and Creamy Chicken

Preparation Time: 5 minutes
Cooking Time: 18 minutes
Servings: 8
Ingredients:

- 4 cups chicken broth
- 2 cups water
- 2 half-cooked and boneless chicken breast, grated
- 1 pack long-grain fast-cooking rice with a spice pack
- 1/2 teaspoon salt
- 1/2 teaspoon ground black pepper
- 3/4 cup flour
- 1/2 cup butter
- 2 cups thick cream

Directions:

1. Combine broth, water, and chicken in a large saucepan over medium heat. Bring to a boil; stir in the rice, and save the seasoning package. Cover and remove from heat.
2. Merge the flour with salt and pepper. Using a medium-sized pan, melt some butter over medium heat. Stir the contents of the herb bag until the mixture bubbles. Reduce the heat and add the flour

mixture to the tablespoon to form a roux. Stir the cream little by little until it is completely absorbed and smooth. Bake until thick for 5 minutes.
3. Add the cream mixture to the stock and rice—cook over medium heat for 10 to 15 minutes.

Nutrition:

- Calories: 462
- Fat: 36.5 g
- Carbohydrates: 22.6 g
- Protein: 12 g

3. Best Spanish rice

Preparation Time: 10 minutes
Cooking Time: 20 minutes
Servings: 5
Ingredients:

- 2 tablespoons oil
- 2 tablespoons chopped onion
- 1 1/2 cups uncooked white rice
- 2 cups chicken broth
- 1 cup chunky salsa

Directions:

1. Heat the oil and stir the onion and cook until tender, about 5 minutes.
2. Mix the rice in a pan, stirring often. When the rice starts to brown, stir in the chicken stock and salsa. Lower the heat, cover, and simmer for 20 minutes until the liquid is absorbed.

Nutrition:

- Calories: 286

- Fat: 6.2 g
- Carbohydrates: 50.9 g
- Protein: 5.7 g

4. Classic Rice Pilaf

Preparation Time: 10 minutes
Cooking Time: 20 minutes
Servings: 6
Ingredients:
- 2 tablespoons butter
- 2 tablespoons olive oil
- 1/2 onion, minced
- 2 cups long-grain white rice
- 3 cups chicken broth
- 1 1/2 teaspoons of salt
- 1 pinch of saffron (optional)
- 1/4 teaspoon of cayenne pepper

Directions:
1. Preheat the oven.
2. Heat the butter until it reaches a liquid form.
3. Attach the melted butter and olive oil to a large saucepan over medium heat.
4. Add and cook the minced onion, continuously stirring until the onion is light brown in color, 7 to 8 minutes. Remove from the heat.
5. Combine rice and onion in a 9x13-inch baking dish on a baking sheet. Mix well to cover the rice.
6. Mix chicken broth, salt, saffron, and cayenne pepper in a pan.

7. Pour the chicken stock mixture over the rice in the casserole and mix. Pour the mixture evenly over the bottom of the pan. Cover firmly with sturdy aluminum foil.
8. Bake and remove from the oven and leave under cover for 10 minutes. Remove the aluminum foil and stir with a fork to separate the rice grains.

Nutrition:

- Calories: 312
- Fat: 9.1 g
- Carbohydrates: 51.7 g
- Protein: 5 g

5. Sarah's Rice Pilaf

Preparation Time: 10 minutes
Cooking Time: 20 minutes
Servings: 4
Ingredients:

- 2 tablespoons butter
- 1/2 cup orzo
- 1/2 cup diced onion
- 2 cloves finely chopped garlic
- 1/2 cup uncooked white rice
- 2 cups chicken broth

Directions:

1. Dissolve the butter in a frying pan. Boil and mix the orzo pasta golden brown.
2. Stir in the onion and cook until it is transparent, then add the garlic and cook for 1 minute.

3. Stir in the rice and chicken broth. Lower the heat until the rice is soft and the liquid is absorbed for 20 to 25 minutes. Detach from heat and let stand for 5 minutes, and then stir with a fork.

Nutrition:

- Calorie 244
- Carbohydrates: 40 g
- Protein: 5.9 g

6. Homemade Fried Rice

Preparation Time: 10 minutes
Cooking Time: 23 minutes
Servings: 8
Ingredients:

- 1 1/2 cup uncooked white rice
- 3 tablespoons sesame oil
- 1 small onion, minced
- 1 clove garlic, minced
- 1 cup peeled shrimp
- 1/2 cup diced ham
- 1 cup chopped cooked chicken fillet
- 2 celery stalks, minced
- 2 carrots, peeled and diced
- 1 green pepper, minced
- 1/2 cup of green peas
- 1 beaten egg
- 1/4 cup soy sauce

Directions:
1. Cook the rice.
2. While cooking the rice, heat a wok or large frying pan over medium heat. Pour in the sesame oil and sauté in the onion until golden brown. Add the garlic, shrimp, ham, and chicken. Cook until the shrimp are pink.
3. Reduce the heat and stir in celery, carrot, green pepper, and peas. Bake until the vegetables are soft. Whip in the beaten egg and cook.
4. When the rice is cooked, merge it with the vegetables and soy sauce.

Nutrition:
- Calories: 236
- Fat: 8.4 g
- Carbohydrates: 26.4 g;
- Protein: 13 g

7. Cranberry Rice

Preparation Time: 5 minutes
Cooking Time: 23 minutes
Servings: 6
Ingredients:
- 2/3 cup uncooked brown rice
- 1 1/2 cups water
- 2 tablespoons canned cranberry sauce
- 1/2 cup of dried cranberries
- Salt and black pepper to taste
- 1/4 cup chopped pecans

Directions:
1. Cook the rice.
2. Squash the cranberry sauce in a small bowl with a fork and mix with the brown rice.
3. Put the dried cranberries in a bowl microwave and cook them on high heat in the microwave for about 30 seconds. Stir the cranberries into the rice. Season it with salt and black pepper; sprinkle with pecans.

Nutrition:
- Calories: 129
- Fat: 3.7 g
- Carbohydrates: 23.4 g
- Protein: 1.6 g

8. Kickin' Rice

Preparation Time: 10 minutes
Cooking Time: 23 minutes
Servings: 6

Ingredients
- 1 tablespoon vegetable oil
- 1 cup long-grain white rice
- 1 can chopped green peppers
- 1 teaspoon ground black pepper
- 2 cups chicken broth

Directions:
1. Heat the vegetable oil. Stir the rice in hot oil.
2. Add the green peppers and keep cooking until the rice starts to turn a little brown, 2 to 3 minutes.

3. Season the rice with pepper. Whisk the stock into the pan; bring to a boil.
4. Reduce the heat to low, cover the pan and cook until the broth has been absorbed.

Nutrition:

- Calories: 83
- Fat: 2.6 g
- Carbohydrates: 13 g
- Protein: 1.9 g

9. Garlic Rice

Preparation Time: 5 minutes
Cooking Time: 15 minutes
Servings: 6
Ingredients:

- 2 tablespoons vegetable oil
- 1 1/2 tablespoons chopped garlic
- 2 tablespoons ground pork
- 4 cups cooked white rice
- 1 1/2 teaspoons of garlic salt
- Ground black pepper to taste

Directions:

1. Heat the oil. Attach the garlic and ground pork. Boil and stir until garlic is golden brown.
2. Stir in cooked white rice and season with garlic, salt, and pepper. Bake and stir until the mixture is hot and well mixed for about 3 minutes.

Nutrition:

- Calories: 83

- Fat: 2.6 g
- Carbohydrates: 13 g
- Protein: 1.9 g

10. Sweet Rice

Preparation Time: 10 minutes
Cooking Time: 15 minutes
Servings: 6
Ingredients:
- 1 cup uncooked long-grain white rice
- 2 tablespoons unsalted butter
- 2 cups water
- 2 cups whole milk
- 1 tablespoon all-purpose flour
- 1/3 cup white sugar
- 1 egg
- 1 1/2 teaspoon vanilla extract
- 1 cup whole milk
- 2/3 cup thick cream
- 1/2 cup raisins (optional)
- 1/2 teaspoon ground cinnamon

Directions:
1. Add rice and butter to water in a large saucepan and bring to boil over high heat.
2. Mix 2 cups of milk, flour, sugar, egg, and vanilla extract in a bowl and pour the milk mixture over the cooked rice. Mix and simmer for 15 minutes over low heat.
3. Stir in 1 cup of whole milk, cream, raisins, and cinnamon until it is well mixed.

Nutrition:

- Calories: 418
- Fat: 18.6 g
- Carbohydrates: 55 g
- Protein: 8.6 g

11. Gourmet Mushroom Risotto

Preparation Time: 20 minutes
Cooking Time: 15 minutes
Servings: 6

Ingredients:

- 1 kg Portobello mushrooms, minced
- 1 pound of white mushrooms, minced
- 2 shallots, diced
- 3 tablespoons olive oil, divided
- 1 1/2 cup Arborio rice
- Salt and black pepper to taste
- 1/2 cup dry white wine
- 4 tablespoons butter
- 3 tablespoons finely chopped chives
- 6 cups chicken broth, divided
- 1/3 cup Parmesan cheese

Directions:

1. Heat the broth over low heat.
2. Attach 2 tablespoons of olive oil in a huge saucepan over medium heat. Whip in the mushrooms and cook until soft. Now remove the mushrooms and their liquid and set them aside.
3. Attach 1 tablespoon of olive oil in the pan and stir in the shallots. Cook for 1 minute and add the rice, stirring, to cover with foil

for about 2 minutes. When the rice has turned a pale golden color, pour the wine constantly, stirring until the wine is completely absorbed.
4. Add 1/2 cup of rice broth and mix until the broth has been absorbed. Continue to add 1/2 cup of broth at a time, constantly stirring.
5. Then detach from the heat and stir in the mushrooms with their liquid, butter, chives, and Parmesan cheese. Season with salt and pepper.

Nutrition:

- Calories: 418
- Fat: 18.6 g
- Carbohydrates: 55 g
- Protein: 8.6 g

12.   John's Beans and Rice

Preparation Time: 20 minutes
Cooking Time: 15 minutes
Servings: 6
Ingredients:

- 1 pound dry red beans
- 1 tablespoon of vegetable oil
- 12 grams of Andouille sausage, diced
- 1 cup finely chopped onion
- 3/4 cup chopped celery
- 3/4 cup poblano peppers
- 4 cloves of garlic, minced
- 2 pints of chicken broth or more if necessary
- 1 smoked ham shank

- 2 bay leaves
- 1 teaspoon dried thyme
- 1/2 teaspoon cayenne pepper
- 1 teaspoon freshly ground black pepper
- 2 tablespoons chopped green onion,
- 4 cups cooked white rice

Directions:
1. Bring the beans in a large container and cover them with a few centimeters of cold water; soak overnight. Drain and rinse.
2. Heat the oil and cook and stir sausage in hot oil for 5 to 7 minutes. Stir in onion, celery, and poblano peppers in sausage; cook and stir until the vegetables soften and start to become transparent, 5 to 10 minutes. Add the garlic to the sausage mixture; cook and stir until fragrant, about 1 minute.
3. Stir in brown beans, chicken broth, ham shank, bay leaf, black pepper, thyme, cayenne pepper, and the sausage mixture; bring to a boil, reduce the heat, and stir occasionally, for an hour and a half.
4. Season with salt and simmer until the beans are soft, the meat is soft, and the desired consistency is achieved, 1 1/2 to 2 hours more. Season with salt.
5. Put the rice in bowls, place the red bean mixture on the rice, and garnish with green onions.

Nutrition:
- Calories: 542
- Fat: 25 g
- Carbohydrates: 36 g
- Protein: 8.6 g

13. Creamy Chicken and Wild Rice Soup

Preparation Time: 10 minutes
Cooking Time: 15 minutes
Servings: 8
Ingredients:
- 2 cups water
- 4 cups chicken broth
- 2 boneless chicken fillet and cooked, grated
- 1 pack long-grain fast-cooking rice with a spice pack
- 1/2 teaspoon salt
- 1/2 teaspoon ground black pepper
- 3/4 cup all-purpose flour
- 1/2 cup butter
- 2 cups thick cream

Directions:
1. Combine broth, water, and chicken in a large saucepan over medium heat. Bring to a boil; stir in the rice, and save the seasoning package. Cover and remove from heat.
2. Merge salt, pepper, and flour. Dissolve the butter. Stir the contents of the herb bag until the mixture bubbles. Reduce the heat and add the flour mixture to a tablespoon to form a roux. Stir the cream little by little until it is completely absorbed and smooth. Bake until thick, 5 minutes.
3. Add the cream mixture to the stock and rice. Cook over medium heat for 10 to 15 minutes.

Nutrition:
- Calories: 426
- Fat: 35 g
- Carbohydrates: 41 g; Protein: 8.6 g

14. Carrot Rice

Preparation Time: 5 minutes
Cooking Time: 15 minutes
Servings: 6
Ingredients:

- 2 cups water
- 1 cube chicken broth
- 1 grated carrot
- 1 cup uncooked long-grain rice

Directions:

1. Boil the water and lace in the bouillon cube and let it dissolve.
2. Stir in the carrots and rice and bring to a boil again.
3. Lower the heats, cover, and simmer for 20 minutes.
4. Remove from heat and leave under cover for 5 minutes.

Nutrition:

- Calories: 125
- Fat: 41 g
- Carbohydrates: 32 g
- Protein: 16 g

15. Rice Sauce

Preparation Time: 5 minutes
Cooking Time: 15 minutes
Servings: 6
Ingredients:

- 3 cups cooked rice
- 1 1/4 cup grated Monterey Jack cheese, divided
- 1 cup canned or frozen corn
- 1/2 cup of milk

- 1/3 cup of sour cream
- 1/2 cup chopped green onions

Directions:
1. Preheat the oven.
2. Combine rice, a cup of cheese, corn, milk, sour cream, and green onions in a medium-sized bowl. Put in a 1-liter baking dish and sprinkle the rest of the cheese over it.
3. Bake until the cheese is dissolved and the dish is hot.

Nutrition:

- Calories: 110
- Fat: 32 g
- Carbohydrates: 54 g
- Protein: 12 g

16. Brown Rice

Preparation Time: 5 minutes
Cooking Time: 15 minutes
Servings: 4
Ingredients:
- 1 1/2 cup white rice
- 1 beef broth
- 1 condensed soup of French onions
- 1/4 cup melted butter
- 1 tablespoon Worcestershire sauce
- 1 tablespoon dried basil leaves

Directions:
1. Preheat the oven.
2. In a 2-quarter oven dish, combine rice, broth, soup, butter, Worcestershire sauce, and basil.

3. Prepare for 1 hour, stirring after 30 minutes.

Nutrition:

- Calories: 425
- Fat: 33 g
- Carbohydrates: 21 g
- Protein: 12 g

17. Rice Lasagna

Preparation Time: 20 minutes
Cooking Time: 15 minutes
Servings: 8
Ingredients:

- 1 pound ground beef
- Spaghetti sauce
- 3 cups cooked rice, cooled
- 1/2 teaspoon garlic powder
- 2 eggs
- 3/4 cup grated Parmesan cheese
- 2 1/4 cup grated mozzarella cheese
- 2 cups of cottage cheese

Directions:

1. Preheat the oven to 190°C.
2. Fry and stir the meat in a hot pan until golden brown and crumbly, 5 to 7 minutes; drain the Fat: and discard it. Add the spaghetti sauce and garlic powder.
3. Mix the rice, eggs, and 1/4 cup Parmesan cheese in a bowl. Mix 2 cups mozzarella, cottage cheese, and 1/4 cup Parmesan cheese in another bowl.

4. Set half of the rice mixture in a 3-liter baking dish, followed by the cheese mixture and half of the meat sauce. Repeat the layers. Sprinkle 1/4 cup Parmesan cheese and 1/4 cup mozzarella on the last layer of meat sauce.
5. Until the cheese is dissolved and the sauce is bubbling 20 to 25 minutes.

Nutrition:

- Calories: 461
- Fat: 31 g
- Carbohydrates: 11 g
- Protein: 13 g

18. Rice Milk

Preparation Time: 5 minutes
Cooking Time: 15 minutes
Servings: 4
Ingredients:
- 4 cups cold water
- 1 cup cooked rice
- 1 teaspoon vanilla extract (optional)

Directions:
1. Combine water, cooked rice, and vanilla extract in a blender; blend until smooth, about 3 minutes.
2. Chill before serving.

Nutrition:

- Calories: 54
- Fat: 32 g
- Carbohydrates: 21 g
- Protein: 26 g

19. Breakfast Salad from Grains and Fruits

Preparation Time: 5 minutes
Cooking Time: 20 minutes
Servings: 6
Ingredients:
- 1/4 teaspoon salt
- 3/4 cup bulgur
- 3/4 cup quick-cooking brown rice
- 1 8-oz low-fat vanilla yogurt
- 1 cup raisins
- 1 Granny Smith apple
- 1 orange
- 1 red delicious apple
- 3 cups water

Directions:
1. On high fire, place a large pot and bring water to a boil.
2. Add bulgur and rice. Slow down the fire to a simmer and cook for ten minutes while covered.
3. Turn off fire, set aside for 2 minutes while covered.
4. On a baking sheet, transfer and evenly spread grains to cool.
5. Meanwhile, peel oranges and cut them into sections. Chop and core apples.
6. Once the grains are cool, transfer to a large serving bowl along with fruits.
7. Add yogurt and mix well to coat.
8. Serve and enjoy.

Nutrition:
- Calories: 48.6; Carbs: 23.9 g ; Protein: 3.7 g ; Fat: 1.1 g

20. Puttanesca Style Bucatini

Preparation Time: 5 minutes
Cooking Time: 40 minutes
Servings: 4
Ingredients:

- 1 tablespoon capers, rinsed
- 1 teaspoon coarsely chopped fresh oregano
- 1 teaspoon finely chopped garlic
- 1/8 teaspoon salt
- 12-oz bucatini pasta
- 2 cups coarsely chopped canned no-salt-added whole peeled tomatoes with their juice
- 3 tablespoons extra virgin olive oil, divided
- 4 anchovy fillets, chopped
- 8 black Kalamata olives, pitted and sliced into slivers

Directions:

1. Cook bucatini pasta according to package directions. Drain, keep warm and set aside.
2. On medium fire, place a large nonstick saucepan and heat 2 tablespoons of oil.
3. Sauté the anchovy until it starts to disintegrate.
4. Add garlic and sauté for 15 seconds.
5. Add tomatoes, sauté for 15 to 20 minutes, or until no longer watery. Season with 1/8 teaspoon salt.
6. Add oregano, capers, and olives.
7. Add pasta, sautéing until heated through.
8. To serve, drizzle pasta with remaining olive oil and enjoy.

Nutrition:

- Calories: 207.4
- Carbs: 31 g
- Protein: 5.1 g
- Fat: 7 g

21. Sausage and Bean Casserole

Preparation Time: 15 minutes
Cooking Time: 45 minutes
Servings: 4
Ingredients:

- 1 pound Italian sausages
- 1 can cannellini beans, drained
- 1 carrot, chopped
- 2 tablespoons olive oil
- 1 onion, chopped
- 2 garlic cloves, minced
- 1 teaspoon paprika
- 1 can tomatoes in juice, chopped
- 1/4 cup chopped fresh parsley
- 1 celery stalk, chopped
- Salt and black pepper to taste

Directions:

1. Preheat oven to 350°F.
2. Heat the olive oil and sauté onion, garlic, celery, and carrot for 3-4 minutes, stirring often until softened. Add in sausages and cook for another 3 minutes, turning occasionally.

3. Stir in paprika for 30 seconds. Turn the heat off and mix in tomatoes, beans, salt, and pepper. Pour into a baking dish and bake for 30 minutes. Serve topped with parsley.

Nutrition:

- Calories: 862
- Fat: 43.6 g
- Carbs: 76.2 g
- Protein: 43.4 g

22. Hot Vegetarian Two-Bean Cassoulet

Preparation Time: 15 minutes
Cooking Time: 40 minutes
Servings: 4
Ingredients:

- 1 cup canned pinto beans, drained
- 1 cup canned can kidney beans, drained
- 2 red bell peppers, seeded and chopped
- 1 onion, chopped
- 1 celery stalk, chopped
- 2 garlic cloves, minced
- 1 can crushed tomatoes
- 2 tablespoons olive oil
- 1 tablespoon red pepper flakes
- 1 teaspoon ground cumin
- Salt and black pepper to taste
- 1/4 teaspoon ground coriander

Directions:

1. Heat the olive oil and sauté bell peppers, celery, garlic, and onion for 5 minutes until tender.

2. Stir in ground cumin, ground coriander, salt, and pepper for 1 minute. Pour in beans, tomatoes, and red pepper flakes. Bring to a boil, then decrease the heat and simmer for another 20 minutes. Serve immediately.

Nutrition:

- Calories: 361
- Fat: 8.4 g
- Carbs: 55.7 g
- Protein: 17.1 g

23. Moroccan Spiced Couscous

Preparation Time: 15 minutes
Cooking Time: 25 minutes
Servings: 4
Ingredients:

- 1 cup instant couscous
- 2 tablespoons dried apricots, chopped
- 2 tablespoons dried sultanas
- 2 tablespoons olive oil
- 1/2 onion, minced
- 1 orange, juiced, and zested
- 1/4 teaspoon paprika
- 1/4 teaspoon turmeric
- 1/2 teaspoon garlic powder
- 1/2 teaspoon ground cumin
- 1/4 teaspoon ground cinnamon
- Salt and black pepper to taste

Directions:
1. Heat the oil and sauté onion for 3 minutes. Add in orange juice, orange zest, garlic powder, cumin, salt, paprika, turmeric, cinnamon, black pepper, and 2 cups of water.
2. Stir in apricots, couscous, and sultanas. Detach from the heat and let it sit for 5 minutes. Fluff the couscous using a fork. Serve.

Nutrition:

- Calories: 246
- Fat: 7.4 g
- Carbs: 41.8 g
- Protein: 5.2 g

24. Bulgur Tabbouleh

Preparation Time: 15 minutes
Cooking Time: 30 minutes
Servings: 4
Ingredients:

- 8 cherry tomatoes, quartered
- 1 cucumber, peeled and chopped
- 1 cup bulgur, rinsed
- 4 scallions, chopped
- 1/2 cup fresh parsley, chopped
- 1 lemon, juiced
- 1/4 cup extra-virgin olive oil
- Salt and black pepper to taste

Directions:
1. Set the bulgur in a large pot with plenty of salted water, cover, and boil for 13-15 minutes. Drain and let it cool completely. Add

scallions, tomatoes, cucumber, and parsley to the cooled bulgur and mix to combine.
2. Merge the lemon juice, olive oil, salt, and pepper. Pour the dressing over the bulgur mixture and toss to combine. Serve chilled.

Nutrition:
- Calories: 291
- Fat: 13.7 g
- Carbs: 40.4 g
- Protein: 7.4 g

25. Parmesan and Collard Green Oats

Preparation Time: 15 minutes
Cooking Time: 15 minutes
Servings: 4
Ingredients:
- 2 cups collard greens, torn into pieces
- 1/2 cup black olives
- 1 cup rolled oats
- 2 tomatoes, diced
- 2 spring onions, chopped
- 1 teaspoon garlic powder
- 1/2 teaspoon hot paprika
- A pinch of salt
- 2 tablespoons fresh parsley, chopped
- 1 tablespoon lemon juice
- 2 tablespoons olive oil
- 1/2 cup Parmesan cheese, grated

Directions:
1. Attach 2 cups of water in a pot over medium heat. Bring to a boil, then lower the heat, and add the rolled oats. Cook for 4-5 minutes.
2. Mix in tomatoes, spring onions, hot paprika, garlic powder, salt, collard greens, black olives, parsley, lemon juice, and olive oil. Cook for another 5 minutes. Spread into bowls and top with Parmesan cheese. Serve warm.

Nutrition:
- Calories: 192
- Fat: 11.2 g
- Carbs: 19.8 g
- Protein: 5.3 g

26. Italian Barley with Artichoke Hearts

Preparation Time: 15 minutes
Cooking Time: 50 minutes
Servings: 4
Ingredients:
- 1 cup pearl barley
- 1/2 cup artichoke hearts, chopped
- 2 tablespoons grated Parmesan cheese
- 1 bay leaf
- 1 fresh cilantro sprig
- 1 fresh thyme sprig
- 2 tablespoons olive oil
- 1 onion, chopped
- 1 tablespoon Italian seasoning
- 3 garlic cloves, minced

- 1 cup chicken broth
- 1 lemon, zested
- Salt and black pepper to taste

Directions:
1. Place barley, cilantro, bay leaf, and thyme in a pot over medium heat and cover with water. Parboil, then lower the heat and simmer for 25 minutes. Drain; discard the bay leaf, rosemary, and thyme and reserve.
2. Heat the olive oil and sauté onion, artichoke, and Italian seasoning for 5 minutes. Add garlic and stir-fry for 40 seconds. Whisk in some broth and cook until the liquid is absorbed, then add more, and keep stirring until it is absorbed again.
3. Mix in lemon zest, salt, pepper, and cheese and stir for 2 minutes until the cheese has melted. Pour over the barley and serve.

Nutrition:
- Calories: 325
- Fat: 12 g
- Carbs: 45.4 g
- Protein: 11.8 g

27. Vegetable Rice Bowl

Preparation Time: 15 minutes
Cooking Time: 25 minutes
Servings: 4
Ingredients:
- 12 ounces broccoli cuts
- 3 cups fresh baby spinach
- 1 red chili, seeded and chopped
- 1 1/2 cups cooked brown rice

- 2 tablespoons olive oil
- 1 onion, chopped
- 1 garlic clove, minced
- 1 orange, juiced, and zested
- 1 cup vegetable broth
- Salt and black pepper to taste

Directions:
1. Heat the oil and sauté onion for 5 minutes, then add in broccoli cuts, and cook for 4-5 minutes until tender. Stir-fry garlic and chili for 30 seconds.
2. Pour in orange zest, orange juice, broth, salt, and pepper, and bring to a boil. Stir in the rice and spinach and cook for 4 minutes until the liquid is reduced. Serve.

Nutrition:

- Calories: 391
- Fat: 9.4 g
- Carbs: 67.6 g
- Protein: 9.8 g

28. Cherry Tomato Rice Pilaf with Pistachios

Preparation Time: 15 minutes
Cooking Time: 30 minutes
Servings: 4
Ingredients:

- 1 cup basmati rice
- 1 carrot, shredded
- 1/2 cup scallions, chopped
- 1 cup cherry tomatoes, halved
- 1 ounce pistachios, crushed

- 2 cups vegetable broth
- 1 garlic clove, minced
- 2 tablespoons olive oil
- 1 teaspoon ground coriander
- 2 tablespoons fresh parsley, chopped

Directions:
1. Heat the oil. Add in the carrot, garlic, and scallions and cook for 3-4 minutes, stirring often. Stir in the rice for 1-2 minutes. Pour in 2 vegetable broths.
2. Bring to a quick boil and sprinkle with ground coriander. Lower the heat and simmer covered for 10-12 minutes until the liquid has been absorbed. Fuzz the rice and transfer it to a serving plate. Top with cherry tomatoes and pistachios and sprinkle with parsley. Serve warm.

Nutrition:

- Calories: 305
- Fat: 11.4 g
- Carbs: 43.8 g
- Protein: 8 g

29. Italian Cannellini Beans with Egg Noodles

Preparation Time: 15 minutes
Cooking Time: 20 minutes
Servings: 4
Ingredients:

- 12 ounces egg noodles
- 1 can diced tomatoes
- 1 can Cannellini beans, drained
- 1/2 cup heavy cream

- 1 cup vegetable stock
- 2 garlic cloves, minced
- 1 onion, chopped
- 3 tablespoons olive oil
- 1 cup spinach, chopped
- 1 teaspoon dill
- 1 teaspoon thyme
- 1/2 teaspoon red pepper, crushed
- 1 lemon, juiced and zested
- 1 tablespoon fresh basil leaves, chopped

Directions:

1. Boil the egg noodles in plenty of salted water for 6 minutes or until al dente. Drain and set aside. Warm the olive oil in a pot over medium heat. Add in onion and garlic and cook for 3 minutes.
2. Stir in dill, thyme, and red pepper for 1 minute.
3. Attach in spinach, vermicelli, vegetable stock, and tomatoes, and parboil.
4. Put in beans and cook until heated through. Combine the heavy cream, lemon juice, lemon zest, and basil. Serve the dish garnished with parsley and the creamy lemon sauce on the side.

Nutrition:

- Calories: 641
- Fat: 19.6 g
- Carbs: 92.1 g
- Protein: 28.7 g

30. Spicy Garbanzo Bowl with Feta Cheese

Preparation Time: 15 minutes

Cooking Time: 10 minutes

Servings: 4

Ingredients:

- 2 cups canned garbanzo beans, drained
- 2 tomatoes, diced
- 1 cucumber, thinly sliced
- 1 teaspoon garlic, minced
- 1 red onion, chopped
- 2 green hot peppers, chopped
- 1 red bell pepper, thinly sliced
- 2 tablespoons fresh parsley, chopped
- 1 fresh lemon, juiced
- 1 cup feta cheese, crumbled
- 1 teaspoon harissa
- 1/4 teaspoon chili flakes
- Salt and black pepper to taste
- Fresh mint leaves, chopped

Directions:

1. Merge the garbanzo beans with cucumber, garlic, onion, hot peppers, tomatoes, bell pepper, parsley, lemon juice, chili flakes, harissa, salt, and black pepper. Adjust the seasonings.
2. Present topped with crumbled feta cheese and freshly chopped mint leaves.

Nutrition:

- Calories: 330
- Fat: 11.6 g
- Carbs: 42.7 g
- Protein: 16.8 g

31. Chickpea and Rice

Preparation Time: 30 min.
Cooking Time: 45 min.
Servings: 4
Ingredients:

- 0.3 lb. long - grain rice, soaked in water for 20 minutes
- 0.3 lb. chickpeas, cooked
- Salt and pepper, to taste
- 1 bay leaf
- 2 tablespoons chopped parsley
- 1 garlic clove minced
- .4 quarts of chicken broth
- 3 tablespoons olive oil
- 1 medium onion, sliced
- 1 teaspoon lime juice

Directions:

1. Drain the rice and set aside.
2. Heat oil in saucepan and cook onion with garlic until onion is softened.
3. Add chickpeas, bay leaf, salt, and pepper. Stir fry for 1-2 minutes.
4. Add chicken broth and let it simmer on medium heat until bubbles appear at the surface.
5. Add rice and lime juice and stir well. Simmer for 4-5 minutes or before the bubbles emerge on the surface or the rice. Now cover the saucepans with a lid and let rice cook on low flame for 20 minutes.
6. Add to serving dish and top with parsley.

7. Serve and enjoy!

Nutrition:

- Calories:321
- Fat:17 g
- Carbs:35 g
- Protein: 21 g

32. One-Pot Rice and Chicken

Preparation Time: 30 min.
Cooking Time: 45 min.
Servings: 4
Ingredients:

- 4-5 chicken thighs
- 0.3 lb. long - grain rice, soaked in water for 20 minutes
- ¼ teaspoons cumin seeds
- 1 teaspoon dried oregano
- Salt and pepper, to taste
- 1 garlic clove, minced
- 0.4 quarts of water
- 3 tablespoons olive oil
- 1 medium onion, sliced
- 1 teaspoon lime juice
- 1 tablespoon vinegar

Directions:

1. In a bowl add chicken, some salt, some black pepper, oregano, cumin, and vinegar. Mix well. Let it marinate for about 20 minutes.

2. Heat some of the oil in the pan and put chicken in the pan.. Let the chicken cook for about 5-6 minutes per side or until nicely golden from both sides. Keep turning the chicken over after a few minutes.
3. Drain the rice and set aside.
4. Preheat oven to 355° F.
5. In a pan, heat some olive oil and cook the onion with garlic until the onion has softened..
6. Add salt and pepper. Stir fry for 1-2 minutes.
7. Add water and let it simmer on medium heat until bubbles appear at the surface.
8. Add rice and lime juice and stir well. Let it simmer for 6-10 minutes or until bubbles appear at the surface or the rice and liquid are dried a little. Place chicken on top of rice.
9. Cover the skillet with a lid and place it in the oven. Bake for 20 minutes.
10. Serve and enjoy!

Nutrition:

- Calories:240
- Fat:15 g
- Carbs:3 g
- Protein: ½ g

33. Grain Bowl with Lentil and Chickpeas

Preparation Time: 10 min.
Cooking Time: 5-8 min.
Servings: 3-4
Ingredients:

- 6 tablespoons virgin olive oil
- Salt, to taste
- 1 zucchini squash, sliced into rounds
- 0.6 lb. farro, cooked
- 0.5 lb. cooked brown lentils, cooked
- ½ lb. chickpeas, cooked
- 0.3 lb. cherry tomatoes, halved
- 2 shallots, sliced
- 2 avocados, peeled, pitted and sliced
- 0.3 lb. fresh parsley, chopped
- 5-6 Kalamata olives
- 2 tablespoons lemon juice
- Some crumbled feta cheese, optional
- 2 tablespoons Dijon mustard
- 1-2 garlic cloves, minced
- 1 teaspoon sumac, ground
- Mixed spices, of choice

Directions:

1. Heat 1-2 tablespoons oil in a pan and sauté zucchini until tender. Removed from heat and set aside.
2. In a bowl add Dijon mustard, some salt, sumac powder, mix spices, remaining olive oil, garlic, and lemon juice; mix well and set aside.
3. Add zucchini, avocado, shallots, farro, lentils, tomatoes, chickpeas, olives, feta, and parsley into serving bowls. Season with Dijon mustard dressing.
4. Serve and enjoy.

Nutrition:

- Calories:625
- Fat: 45 g
- Carbs: 0 g
- Protein: 15 g

34. White Beans with Vegetables

Preparation Time: 10 min.
Cooking Time: 0 min.
Servings: 4
Ingredients:

- ½ lb. white beans, cooked
- 1 onion, chopped
- 1 tablespoon lemon juice
- 7-8 cherry tomatoes, chopped
- 1 tablespoon oregano
- Ground pepper, to taste
- 2-3 tablespoons cilantro, chopped
- Salt, to taste

Directions:

1. In a large bowl combine white beans, onion, tomatoes, cilantro, oregano, salt, pepper, and lemon juice.
2. Add mixture to a serving dish.
3. Enjoy.

Nutrition:

- Calories: 345
- Fat: 27 g
- Carbs: 67 g
- Protein: 21 g

35. Yangchow Chinese Style Fried Rice

Preparation Time: 5 minutes
Cooking Time: 20 minutes
Servings: 4

Ingredients:

- 4 cups cold cooked rice
- 1/2 cup peas
- 1 medium yellow onion, diced
- 5 tbsp olive oil
- 4 oz frozen medium shrimp, thawed, shelled, deveined and chopped finely
- 6 oz roast pork
- 3 large eggs
- Salt and freshly ground black pepper
- 1/2 tsp cornstarch

Directions:

1. Combine the salt and ground black pepper and 1/2 tsp cornstarch, coat the shrimp with it. Chop the roasted pork. Beat the eggs and set aside.
2. Stir-fry the shrimp in a wok on high fire with 1 tbsp heated oil until pink, around 3 minutes. Set the shrimp aside and stir fry the roasted pork briefly. Remove both from the pan.

3. In the same pan, stir-fry the onion until soft, Stir the peas and cook until bright green. Remove both from pan.
4. Add 2 tbsp oil in the same pan, add the cooked rice. Stir and separate the individual grains. Add the beaten eggs, toss the rice. Add the roasted pork, shrimp, vegetables and onion. Toss everything together. Season with salt and pepper to taste.

Nutrition:

- Calories: 556
- Carbs: 60.2g
- Protein: 20.2g
- Fat: 25.2g

36. Seafood and Veggie Pasta

Preparation Time: 5 minutes
Cooking Time: 20 minutes
Servings: 4
Ingredients:

- ¼ tsp pepper
- ¼ tsp salt
- 1 lb raw shelled shrimp
- 1 lemon, cut into wedges
- 1 tbsp butter
- 1 tbsp olive oil
- 2 5-oz cans chopped clams, drained (reserve 2 tbsp clam juice)
- 2 tbsp dry white wine
- 4 cloves garlic, minced
- 4 cups zucchini, spiraled (use a veggie spiralizer)
- 4 tbsp Parmesan Cheese

- Chopped fresh parsley to garnish

Directions:

1. Ready the zucchini and spiralize with a veggie spiralizer. Arrange 1 cup of zucchini noodle per bowl. Total of 4 bowls.
2. On medium fire, place a large nonstick saucepan and heat oil and butter.
3. For a minute, sauté garlic. Add shrimp and cook for 3 minutes until opaque or cooked.
4. Add white wine, reserved clam juice and clams. Bring to a simmer and continue simmering for 2 minutes or until half of liquid has evaporated. Stir constantly.
5. Season with pepper and salt. And if needed add more to taste.
6. Remove from fire and evenly distribute seafood sauce to 4 bowls.
7. Top with a tablespoonful of Parmesan cheese per bowl, serve and enjoy.

Nutrition:

- Calories: 324.9
- Carbs: 12g
- Protein: 43.8g
- Fat: 11.3g

37. Seafood Paella with Couscous

Preparation Time: 5 minutes
Cooking Time: 15 minutes
Servings: 4
Ingredients:

- ½ cup whole wheat couscous

- 4 oz small shrimp, peeled and deveined
- 4 oz bay scallops, tough muscle removed
- ¼ cup vegetable broth
- 1 cup freshly diced tomatoes and juice
- Pinch of crumbled saffron threads
- ¼ tsp freshly ground pepper
- ¼ tsp salt
- ½ tsp fennel seed
- ½ tsp dried thyme
- 1 clove garlic, minced
- 1 medium onion, chopped
- 2 tsp extra virgin olive oil

Directions:

1. Put on medium fire a large saucepan and add oil. Stir in the onion and sauté for three minutes before adding: saffron, pepper, salt, fennel seed, thyme, and garlic. Continue to sauté for another minute.
2. Then add the broth and tomatoes and let boil. Once boiling, reduce the fire, cover and continue to cook for another 2 minutes.
3. Add the scallops and increase fire to medium and stir occasionally and cook for two minutes. Add the shrimp and wait for two minutes more before adding the couscous. Then remove from fire, cover and set aside for five minutes before carefully mixing.

Nutrition:

- Calories: 117
- Carbs: 11.7g

- Protein: 11.5g
- Fat: 3.1g

38. Shrimp Paella Made with Quinoa

Preparation Time: 10 minutes
Cooking Time: 40 minutes
Servings: 7
Ingredients:

- 1 lb. large shrimp, peeled, deveined and thawed
- 1 tsp seafood seasoning
- 1 cup frozen green peas
- 1 red bell pepper, cored, seeded & membrane removed, sliced into ½" strips
- ½ cup sliced sun-dried tomatoes, packed in olive oil
- Salt to taste
- ½ tsp black pepper
- ½ tsp Spanish paprika
- ½ tsp saffron threads (optional turmeric)
- 1 bay leaf
- ¼ tsp crushed red pepper flakes
- 3 cups chicken broth, fat free, low sodium
- 1 ½ cups dry quinoa, rinse well
- 1 tbsp olive oil
- 2 cloves garlic, minced
- 1 yellow onion, diced

Directions:

1. Season shrimps with seafood seasoning and a pinch of salt. Toss to mix well and refrigerate until ready to use.

2. Prepare and wash quinoa. Set aside.
3. On medium low fire, place a large nonstick skillet and heat oil. Add onions and for 5 minutes sauté until soft and tender.
4. Add paprika, saffron (or turmeric), bay leaves, red pepper flakes, chicken broth and quinoa. Season with salt and pepper.
5. Cover skillet and bring to a boil. Once boiling, lower fire to a simmer and cook until all liquid is absorbed, around ten minutes.
6. Add shrimp, peas and sun-dried tomatoes. For 5 minutes, cover and cook.
7. Once done, turn off fire and for ten minutes allow paella to set while still covered.
8. To serve, remove bay leaf and enjoy with a squeeze of lemon if desired.

Nutrition:

- Calories: 324.4
- Protein: 22g
- Carbs: 33g;
- Fat: 11.6g

39. Shrimp, Lemon and Basil Pasta

Preparation Time: 5 minutes
Cooking Time: 25 minutes
Servings: 4
Ingredients:

- 2 cups baby spinach
- ½ tsp salt
- 2 tbsp fresh lemon juice
- 2 tbsp extra virgin olive oil

- 3 tbsp drained capers
- ¼ cup chopped fresh basil
- 1 lb. peeled and deveined large shrimp
- 8 oz uncooked spaghetti
- 3 quarts water

Directions:

1. In a pot, bring to boil 3 quarts water. Add the pasta and allow to boil for another eight mins before adding the shrimp and simmering for another three mins or until pasta is cooked.
2. Drain the pasta and transfer to a bowl. Add salt, lemon juice, olive oil, capers and basil while mixing well.
3. To serve, place baby spinach on plate around ½ cup and topped with ½ cup of pasta.

Nutrition: Calories: 151; Carbs: 18.9g; Protein: 4.3g; Fat: 7.4g

40. Simple Penne Anti-Pasto

Preparation Time: 5 minutes
Cooking Time: 15 minutes
Servings: 4
Ingredients:

- ¼ cup pine nuts, toasted
- ½ cup grated Parmigiano-Reggiano cheese, divided
- 8oz penne pasta, cooked and drained
- 1 6oz jar drained, sliced, marinated and quartered artichoke hearts
- 1 7 oz jar drained and chopped sun-dried tomato halves packed in oil
- 3 oz chopped prosciutto

- 1/3 cup pesto
- ½ cup pitted and chopped Kalamata olives
- 1 medium red bell pepper

Directions:

1. Slice bell pepper, discard membranes, seeds and stem. On a foiled lined baking sheet, place bell pepper halves, press down by hand and broil in oven for eight minutes. Remove from oven, put in a sealed bag for 5 minutes before peeling and chopping.
2. Place chopped bell pepper in a bowl and mix in artichokes, tomatoes, prosciutto, pesto and olives.
3. Toss in ¼ cup cheese and pasta. Transfer to a serving dish and garnish with ¼ cup cheese and pine nuts. Serve and enjoy!

Nutrition: Calories: 606; Carbs: 70.3g; Protein: 27.2g; Fat: 27.6g

41. Spaghetti in Lemon Avocado White Sauce

Preparation Time: 5 minutes
Cooking Time: 30 minutes
Servings: 6
Ingredients:

- Freshly ground black pepper
- Zest and juice of 1 lemon
- 1 avocado, pitted and peeled
- 1-pound spaghetti
- Salt
- 1 tbsp Olive oil
- 8 oz small shrimp, shelled and deveined
- ¼ cup dry white wine
- 1 large onion, finely sliced

Directions:

1. Let a big pot of water boil. Once boiling add the spaghetti or pasta and cook following manufacturer's instructions until al dente. Drain and set aside.
2. In a large fry pan, over medium fire sauté wine and onions for ten minutes or until onions are translucent and soft.
3. Add the shrimps into the fry pan and increase fire to high while constantly sautéing until shrimps are cooked around five minutes. Turn the fire off. Season with salt and add the oil right away. Then quickly toss in the cooked pasta, mix well.
4. In a blender, until smooth, puree the lemon juice and avocado. Pour into the fry pan of pasta, combine well. Garnish with pepper and lemon zest then serve.

Nutrition:

- Calories: 206
- Carbs: 26.3g
- Protein: 10.2g
- Fat: 8.0g

42. Spanish Rice Casserole with Cheesy Beef

Preparation Time: 5 minutes
Cooking Time: 32 minutes
Servings: 2
Ingredients:

- 2 tablespoons chopped green bell pepper
- 1/4 teaspoon Worcestershire sauce
- 1/4 teaspoon ground cumin
- 1/4 cup shredded Cheddar cheese

- 1/4 cup finely chopped onion
- 1/4 cup chile sauce
- 1/3 cup uncooked long grain rice
- 1/2-pound lean ground beef
- 1/2 teaspoon salt
- 1/2 teaspoon brown sugar
- 1/2 pinch ground black pepper
- 1/2 cup water
- 1/2 (14.5 ounce) can canned tomatoes
- 1 tablespoon chopped fresh cilantro

Directions:

1. Place a nonstick saucepan on medium fire and brown beef for 10 minutes while crumbling beef. Discard fat.
2. Stir in pepper, Worcestershire sauce, cumin, brown sugar, salt, chile sauce, rice, water, tomatoes, green bell pepper, and onion. Mix well and cook for 10 minutes until blended and a bit tender.
3. Transfer to an ovenproof casserole and press down firmly. Sprinkle cheese on top and cook for 7 minutes at 400oF preheated oven. Broil for 3 minutes until top is lightly browned.
4. Serve and enjoy with chopped cilantro.

Nutrition:

- Calories: 460
- Carbohydrates: 35.8g
- Protein: 37.8g
- Fat: 17.9g

43. Squash and Eggplant Casserole

Preparation Time: 5 minutes
Cooking Time: 45 minutes
Servings: 2
Ingredients:

- ½ cup dry white wine
- 1 eggplant, halved and cut to 1-inch slices
- 1 large onion, cut into wedges
- 1 red bell pepper, seeded and cut to julienned strips
- 1 small butternut squash, cut into 1-inch slices
- 1 tbsp olive oil
- 12 baby corn
- 2 cups low sodium vegetable broth
- Salt and pepper to taste
- Polenta Ingredients
- ¼ cup parmesan cheese, grated
- 1 cup instant polenta
- 2 tbsp fresh oregano, chopped
- Topping Ingredients
- 1 garlic clove, chopped
- 2 tbsp slivered almonds
- 5 tbsp parsley, chopped
- Grated zest of 1 lemon

Directions:

1. Preheat the oven to 350 degrees Fahrenheit.
2. In a casserole, heat the oil and add the onion wedges and baby corn. Sauté over medium high heat for five minutes. Stir

occasionally to prevent the onions and baby corn from sticking at the bottom of the pan.
3. Add the butternut squash to the casserole and toss the vegetables. Add the eggplants and the red pepper.
4. Cover the vegetables and cook over low to medium heat.
5. Cook for about ten minutes before adding the wine. Let the wine sizzle before stirring in the broth. Bring to a boil and cook in the oven for 30 minutes.
6. While the casserole is cooking inside the oven, make the topping by spreading the slivered almonds on a baking tray and toasting under the grill until they are lightly browned.
7. Place the toasted almonds in a small bowl and mix the remaining ingredients for the toppings.
8. Prepare the polenta. In a large saucepan, bring 3 cups of water to boil over high heat.
9. Add the polenta and continue whisking until it absorbs all the water.
10. Reduce the heat to medium until the polenta is thick. Add the parmesan cheese and oregano.
11. Serve the polenta on plates and add the casserole on top. Sprinkle the toppings on top.

Nutrition: Calories: 579.3; Carbs: 79.2g; Protein: 22.2g; Fat: 19.3g

44. Stuffed Tomatoes with Green Chili

Preparation Time: 5 minutes
Cooking Time: 55 minutes
Servings: 2
Ingredients:

- 4 oz Colby-Jack shredded cheese

- ¼ cup water
- 1 cup uncooked quinoa
- 6 large ripe tomatoes
- ¼ tsp freshly ground black pepper
- ¾ tsp ground cumin
- 1 tsp salt, divided
- 1 tbsp fresh lime juice
- 1 tbsp olive oil
- 1 tbsp chopped fresh oregano
- 1 cup chopped onion
- 2 cups fresh corn kernels
- 2 poblano chilies

Directions:

1. Preheat broiler to high.
2. Slice lengthwise the chilies and press on a baking sheet lined with foil. Broil for 8 minutes. Remove from oven and let cool for 10 minutes. Peel the chilies and chop coarsely and place in medium sized bowl.
3. Place onion and corn in baking sheet and broil for ten minutes. Stir two times while broiling. Remove from oven and mix in with chopped chilies.
4. Add black pepper, cumin, ¼ tsp salt, lime juice, oil and oregano. Mix well.
5. Cut off the tops of tomatoes and set aside. Leave the tomato shell intact as you scoop out the tomato pulp.
6. Drain tomato pulp as you press down with a spoon. Reserve 1 ¼ cups of tomato pulp liquid and discard the rest. Invert the tomato shells on a wire rack for 30 mins and then wipe the insides dry with a paper towel.

7. Season with ½ tsp salt the tomato pulp.
8. On a sieve over a bowl, place quinoa. Add water until it covers quinoa. Rub quinoa grains for 30 seconds together with hands; rinse and drain. Repeat this procedure two times and drain well at the end.
9. In medium saucepan bring to a boil remaining salt, ¼ cup water, quinoa and tomato liquid.
10. Once boiling, reduce heat and simmer for 15 minutes or until liquid is fully absorbed. Remove from heat and fluff quinoa with fork. Transfer and mix well the quinoa with the corn mixture.
11. Spoon ¾ cup of the quinoa-corn mixture into the tomato shells, top with cheese and cover with the tomato top. Bake in a preheated 350oF oven for 15 minutes and then broil high for another 1.5 minutes.

Nutrition:

- Calories: 276
- Carbs: 46.3g
- Protein: 13.4g
- Fat: 4.1g

45. Tasty Lasagna Rolls

Preparation Time: 5 minutes
Cooking Time: 20 minutes
Servings: 2
Ingredients:

- ¼ tsp crushed red pepper
- ¼ tsp salt
- ½ cup shredded mozzarella cheese

- ½ cups parmesan cheese, shredded
- 1 14-oz package tofu, cubed
- 1 25-oz can of low-sodium marinara sauce
- 1 tbsp extra virgin olive oil
- 12 whole wheat lasagna noodles
- 2 tbsp Kalamata olives, chopped
- 3 cloves minced garlic
- 3 cups spinach, chopped

Directions:

1. Put enough water on a large pot and cook the lasagna noodles according to package instructions. Drain, rinse and set aside until ready to use.
2. In a large skillet, sauté garlic over medium heat for 20 seconds. Add the tofu and spinach and cook until the spinach wilts. Transfer this mixture in a bowl and add parmesan olives, salt, red pepper and 2/3 cup of the marinara sauce.
3. In a pan, spread a cup of marinara sauce on the bottom. To make the rolls, place noodle on a surface and spread ¼ cup of the tofu filling. Roll up and place it on the pan with the marinara sauce. Do this procedure until all lasagna noodles are rolled.
4. Place the pan over high heat and bring to a simmer. Reduce the heat to medium and let it cook for three more minutes. Sprinkle mozzarella cheese and let the cheese melt for two minutes. Serve hot.

Nutrition:

- Calories: 304
- Carbs: 39.2g
- Protein: 23g; Fat: 19.2g

46. Tasty Mushroom Bolognese

Preparation Time: 10 minutes
Cooking Time: 65 minutes
Servings: 6
Ingredients:

- ¼ cup chopped fresh parsley
- oz Parmigiano-Reggiano cheese, grated
- 1 tbsp kosher salt
- 10-oz whole wheat spaghetti, cooked and drained
- ¼ cup milk
- 1 14-oz can whole peeled tomatoes
- ½ cup white wine
- 2 tbsp tomato paste
- 1 tbsp minced garlic
- 8 cups finely chopped cremini mushrooms
- ½ lb. ground pork
- ½ tsp freshly ground black pepper, divided
- ¾ tsp kosher salt, divided
- 2 ½ cups chopped onion
- 1 tbsp olive oil
- 1 cup boiling water
- ½-oz dried porcini mushrooms

Directions:

1. Let porcini stand in a boiling bowl of water for twenty minutes, drain (reserve liquid), rinse and chop. Set aside.
2. On medium high fire, place a Dutch oven with olive oil and cook for ten minutes cook pork, ¼ tsp pepper, ¼ tsp salt and onions. Constantly mix to break ground pork pieces.

3. Stir in ¼ tsp pepper, ¼ tsp salt, garlic and cremini mushrooms. Continue cooking until liquid has evaporated, around fifteen minutes.
4. Stirring constantly, add porcini and sauté for a minute.
5. Stir in wine, porcini liquid, tomatoes and tomato paste. Let it simmer for forty minutes. Stir occasionally. Pour milk and cook for another two minutes before removing from fire.
6. Stir in pasta and transfer to a serving dish. Garnish with parsley and cheese before serving.

Nutrition:

- Calories: 358
- Carbs: 32.8g
- Protein: 21.1g
- Fat: 15.4g

47. Tortellini Salad with Broccoli

Preparation Time: 10 minutes
Cooking Time: 20 minutes
Servings: 12
Ingredients:

- 1 red onion, chopped finely
- 1 cup sunflower seeds
- 1 cup raisins
- 3 heads fresh broccoli, cut into florets
- 2 tsp cider vinegar
- ½ cup white sugar
- ½ cup mayonnaise
- 20-oz fresh cheese filled tortellini

Directions:

1. In a large pot of boiling water, cook tortellini according to manufacturer's instructions. Drain and rinse with cold water and set aside.
2. Whisk vinegar, sugar and mayonnaise to create your salad dressing.
3. Mix together in a large bowl red onion, sunflower seeds, raisins, tortellini and broccoli. Pour dressing and toss to coat.
4. Serve and enjoy.

Nutrition: Calories: 272; Carbs: 38.7g; Protein: 5.0g; Fat: 8.1g

48. Turkey and Quinoa Stuffed Peppers

Preparation Time: 5 minutes
Cooking Time: 55 minutes
Servings: 6
Ingredients:

- 3 large red bell peppers
- 2 tsp chopped fresh rosemary
- 2 tbsp chopped fresh parsley
- 3 tbsp chopped pecans, toasted
- ¼ cup extra virgin olive oil
- ½ cup chicken stock
- ½ lb. fully cooked smoked turkey sausage, diced
- ½ tsp salt
- 2 cups water
- 1 cup uncooked quinoa

Directions:

1. On high fire, place a large saucepan and add salt, water and quinoa. Bring to a boil.
2. Once boiling, reduce fire to a simmer, cover and cook until all water is absorbed around 15 minutes.
3. Uncover quinoa, turn off fire and let it stand for another 5 minutes.
4. Add rosemary, parsley, pecans, olive oil, chicken stock and turkey sausage into pan of quinoa. Mix well.
5. Slice peppers lengthwise in half and discard membranes and seeds. In another boiling pot of water, add peppers, boil for 5 minutes, drain and discard water.
6. Grease a 13 x 9 baking dish and preheat oven to 350oF.
7. Place boiled bell pepper onto prepared baking dish, evenly fill with the quinoa mixture and pop into oven.
8. Bake for 15 minutes.

Nutrition:

- Calories: 255.6
- Carbs: 21.6g
- Protein: 14.4g
- Fat: 12.4g

49. Veggie Pasta with Shrimp, Basil and Lemon

Preparation Time: 5 minutes
Cooking Time: 5 minutes
Servings: 4
Ingredients:

- 2 cups baby spinach
- ½ tsp salt

- 2 tbsp fresh lemon juice
- 2 tbsp extra virgin olive oil
- 3 tbsp drained capers
- ¼ cup chopped fresh basil
- 1 lb. peeled and deveined large shrimp
- 4 cups zucchini, spirals

Directions:

1. divide into 4 serving plates, top with ¼ cup of spinach, serve and enjoy.

Nutrition:

- Calories: 51
- Carbs: 4.4g
- Protein: 1.8g
- Fat: 3.4g

50. Veggies and Sun-Dried Tomato Alfredo

Preparation Time: 5 minutes
Cooking Time: 30 minutes
Servings: 4
Ingredients:

- 2 tsp finely shredded lemon peel
- ½ cup finely shredded Parmesan cheese
- 1 ¼ cups milk
- 2 tbsp all-purpose flour
- 8 fresh mushrooms, sliced
- 1 ½ cups fresh broccoli florets
- 4 oz fresh trimmed and quartered Brussels sprouts

- 4 oz trimmed fresh asparagus spears
- 1 tbsp olive oil
- 4 tbsp butter
- ½ cup chopped dried tomatoes
- 8 oz dried fettuccine

Directions:

1. In a boiling pot of water, add fettuccine and cook following manufacturer's instructions. Two minutes before the pasta is cooked, add the dried tomatoes. Drain pasta and tomatoes and return to pot to keep warm. Set aside.
2. On medium high fire, in a big fry pan with 1 tbsp butter, fry mushrooms, broccoli, Brussels sprouts and asparagus. Cook for eight minutes while covered, transfer to a plate and put aside.
3. Using same fry pan, add remaining butter and flour. Stirring vigorously, cook for a minute or until thickened. Add Parmesan cheese, milk and mix until cheese is melted around five minutes.
4. Toss in the pasta and mix. Transfer to serving dish. Garnish with Parmesan cheese and lemon peel before serving.

Nutrition:

- Calories: 439
- Carbs: 52.0g
- Protein:16.3g
- Fat: 19.5g

Chapter 2. Desserts

1. Dessert Pie

Preparation Time: 10 minutes
Cooking Time: 18 minutes
Servings: 12
Ingredients:
- 1/3 cup all-purpose flour
- 1 package of cream cheese
- 8 ounces whipped cream topping
- 1 package of instant chocolate pudding
- 1/2 cup butter, white sugar

Directions:
1. Preheat the oven.
2. Merge the butter, flour, and 1/4 cup sugar until the mixture looks like coarse breadcrumbs. Bake until lightly browned to allow cooling to room temperature.
3. Whip cream cheese and 1/2 cup sugar until smooth. Stir in half of the whipped topping. Spread the mixture over the cooled crust.
4. Mix the pudding in the same bowl according to the instructions on the package. Spread over the cream cheese mixture.
5. Garnish with the remaining whipped cream. Cool in the fridge.

Nutrition:
- Calories: 376
- Fat: 23 g
- Protein: 3.6 g

2. Date Balls

Preparation Time: 10 minutes
Cooking Time: 5 minutes
Servings: 1
Ingredients:
- 3/4 cup walnuts
- 12 Medjool dates
- 1/2 cup butter
- 1 cup pistachios
- 1 cup coconut flakes

Directions:
1. Preheat the oven.
2. Whip walnuts on a baking sheet, and toast for 5 minutes.
3. Merge the toasted walnuts for 30 seconds or until evenly ground. Transfer walnuts to a medium bowl.
4. In the food processor, blend Medjool dates and butter for 2 minutes until the mixture resembles a paste.
5. Merge the walnuts and date paste.
6. Place ground pistachios, and place coconut flakes in a separate small bowl.
7. Set and present each date ball in a mini cupcake liner, serve.

Nutrition:
- Calories: 212
- Fat: 25 g
- Protein: 3.6 g

3. Sugar-coated Pecans

Preparation Time: 10 minutes
Cooking Time: 1 hour

Servings: 12
Ingredients:
- 1 egg white
- 1 tablespoon water
- 1-pound pecan halves
- 1 cup white sugar
- 1/2 teaspoon ground cinnamon

Directions:
1. Preheat the oven.

Merge the egg whites and water until frothy. Combine the sugar, add to the ingredients list, and cinnamon in another bowl.

2. Attach the pecans to the egg whites and stir to cover the nuts. Remove the nuts and mix them with the sugar until well covered.
3. Bake for 1 hour and whisk every 15 minutes.

Nutrition:
- Calories: 328
- Fat: 27.2 g
- Protein: 3.8 g

4. Jalapeño Popper Spread

Preparation Time: 10 minutes
Cooking Time: 3 minutes
Servings: 32
Ingredients:
- 2 packets of cream cheese, softened
- 1/2 cup mayonnaise
- 1 (4-gram) can chopped green peppers, drained
- grams diced jalapeño peppers, canned, drained

- 1 cup grated Parmesan cheese

Directions:
1. Merge the cream cheese and mayonnaise until smooth. Stir the bell peppers and jalapeño peppers.
2. Pour the mixture into a microwave oven and sprinkle with Parmesan cheese.
3. Microwave on maximum power, about 3 minutes.

Nutrition:
- Calories: 110
- Fat: 11.1 g
- Protein: 2.1 g

5. Delicious French Eclairs

Preparation Time: 10 minutes
Cooking Time: 43 minutes
Servings: 12
Ingredients:
- 1/2 cup butter
- 1 cup boiling water
- 1 cup sifted flour
- 4 eggs
- A pinch of salt

Directions:
1. In a medium saucepan, combine butter, salt, and boiling water. Bring to the boil, then reduce heat and add a cup of flour all at once.
2. Detach from heat and attach eggs, one at a time, whisking well to incorporate completely after each addition.

3. Spoon onto a lined baking sheet, then bake for 20 minutes in a preheated to 450°F oven. Reduce heat to 350°F and bake for 20 minutes more or until golden. Set aside to cool and fill with sweetened whipped cream or custard.

Nutrition:
- Calories: 220
- Fat: 17 g
- Protein: 5 g

6. Sweet Tropical Medley Smoothie

Preparation Time: 10 minutes
Cooking Time: 5 minutes
Servings: 4
Ingredients:
- 1 banana, peeled
- 1 sliced mango
- 1 cup fresh pineapple
- 1/2 cup coconut water

Directions:
1. Place all in a blender.
2. Blend until smooth.
3. Whip in a glass container and allow chilling in the fridge for at least 30 minutes.

Nutrition:
- Calories: 73
- Carbs: 18.6 g
- Protein: 0.8 g
- Fat: 0.5 g

7. Ginger Pineapple

Preparation Time: 10 minutes
Cooking Time: 5 minutes
Servings: 4
Ingredients:
- 10 ounces fresh pineapple
- 1/2 teaspoon ground ginger
- 1 tablespoon almond butter, softened

Directions:
1. Slice the pineapple into the serving pieces and brush with almond butter.
2. After this, sprinkle every pineapple piece with ground ginger.
3. Preheat the grill to 400°F.
4. Grill the pineapple for 2 minutes from each side.
5. The cooked fruit should have a light brown surface on both sides.

Nutrition:
- Calories: 61 g
- Fat: 2.4 g
- Fiber: 1.4 g
- Carbs: 10.2 g
- Protein: 1.3 g

8. Roasted Berry and Honey Yogurt Pops

Preparation Time: 8 minutes
Cooking Time: 15 minutes
Servings: 4
Ingredients:
- 12 ounces mixed berries

- A dash of sea salt
- 2 tablespoons honey
- 2 cups whole Greek yogurt
- 1/2 small lemon, juice

Directions:
1. Preheat the oven.
2. Merge the berries with sea salt and honey.
3. Pour the berries on the prepared baking sheet.
4. Roast for 30 minutes while stirring halfway.
5. While the fruit is roasting, blend the Greek yogurt and lemon juice. Add honey to taste if desired.
6. Once the berries are done, cool for at least ten minutes.
7. Fold the berries into the yogurt mixture.
8. Serve chilled.

Nutrition:
- Calories: 177
- Carbs: 24.8 g
- Protein: 3.2 g
- Fat: 7.9 g

9. Key Lime Pie

Preparation Time: 8 minutes
Cooking Time: 9 minutes
Servings: 8
Ingredients:
- 9-inch prepared graham cracker crust
- 2 cups of sweetened condensed milk
- 1/2 cup sour cream
- 3/4 cup lime juice

- 1 tablespoon grated lime zest

Directions:
1. Preheat the oven.
2. Combine the condensed milk, sour cream, lime juice, and lime zest in a medium bowl. Merge well and pour into the graham cracker crust.
3. Bake in the preheated oven for 5 to 8 minutes until small bubbles burst on the surface of the cake.
4. Cool the cake well before serving. Decorate with lime slices and whipped cream if desired.

Nutrition:
- Calories: 553
- Fat: 20.5 g
- Protein: 10.9 g

10. Healthy Zucchini Pudding

Preparation Time: 8 minutes
Cooking Time: 10 minutes
Servings: 4
Ingredients:
- 2 cups zucchini, shredded
- 1/4 teaspoon cardamom powder
- 5 ounces half and half
- 5 ounces almond milk
- 1/4 cup Swerve

Directions:
1. Add all ingredients except cardamom into the instant pot and stir well.

   Seal the pot with the lid and cook on high.

2. Release pressure gently for 10 minutes, then release remaining using quick release. Remove the lid.
3. Stir in cardamom and serve.

Nutrition:
- Calories: 137
- Fat: 12.6 g
- Carbohydrates: 20.5 g
- Protein: 2.6 g

11. Chocolate Ganache

Preparation Time: 8 minutes
Cooking Time: 3 minutes
Servings: 16
Ingredients:
- 9 ounces bittersweet chocolate, chopped
- 1/2 cup heavy cream
- 1 tablespoon dark rum (optional)

Directions:
1. Place the chocolate in a medium bowl. Heat the cream in a small saucepan.
2. Bring to a boil. When the cream has reached a boiling point, pour the chopped chocolate over it and beat until smooth. Stir the rum if desired.
3. Allow the ganache to cool slightly before you pour it on a cake. Begin in the middle of the cake and work outside. For a fluffy icing or chocolate filling, let it cool until thick and beat with a whisk until light and fluffy.

Nutrition:
- Calories: 137
- Fat: 12.6 g
- Carbohydrates: 20.5 g
- Protein: 2.6 g

12. Simple Peanut Butter and Chocolate Balls

Preparation Time: 8 minutes
Cooking Time: 0 minutes
Servings: 15
Ingredients:
- 3/4 cup creamy peanut butter
- 1/4 cup unsweetened cocoa powder
- 2 tablespoons softened almond butter
- 1/2 teaspoon vanilla extract
- 1 3/4 cups maple sugar

Directions:
1. Line a baking sheet with parchment paper.
2. Combine all the ingredients in a bowl. Stir to mix well.
3. Divide the mixture into 15 parts and shape each part into a 1-inch ball.
4. Arrange the balls on the baking sheet and refrigerate for at least 30 minutes, then serve chilled.

Nutrition:
- Calories: 146
- Fat: 8.1 g
- Protein: 4.2 g

13. Mango Bowls

Preparation Time: 5 minutes
Cooking Time: 0 minutes
Servings: 4
Ingredients:
- 3 cups mango, cut into medium chunks
- 1/2 cup coconut water
- 1/4 cup stevia
- 1 teaspoon vanilla extract

Directions:
1. Merge the mango with the rest of the ingredients, pulse well, divide into bowls, and serve cold.

Nutrition:
- Calories: 122
- Fat: 4 g
- Fiber: 5.3 g
- Carbs: 6.6 g
- Protein: 4.5 g

14. Walnut Apple Pear Mix

Preparation Time: 4 minutes
Cooking Time: 0 minutes
Servings: 4
Ingredients:
- 2 apples, cored and cut into wedges
- 1/2 teaspoon vanilla
- 1 cup apple juice
- 2 tablespoons walnuts, chopped
- 2 apples, cored and cut into wedges

Directions:
1. Attach all ingredients into the inner pot of the instant pot and stir well.
2. Seal pot with lid and cook on high.
3. Set pressure naturally, then release remaining using quick release. Remove lid.
4. Serve and enjoy.

Nutrition:
- Calories: 132
- Fat: 2.6 g
- Carbohydrates: 28.3 g
- Sugar: 21.9 g
- Protein: 1.3 g
- Cholesterol: 0 mg

15. Spiced Pear Sauce

Preparation Time: 4 minutes
Cooking Time: 6 hours
Servings: 12
Ingredients:
- 8 pears, cored and diced
- 1/2 teaspoon ground cinnamon
- 1/4 teaspoon ground nutmeg
- 1/4 teaspoon ground cardamom
- 1 cup of water

Directions:
1. Attach all ingredients into the instant pot and stir well.
2. Seal the pot with a lid and select slow cook mode and cook on low for 6 hours.

3. Mash the sauce using a potato masher.
4. Whip into the container and freeze it in the fridge.

Nutrition:
- Calories: 81
- Fat: 0.2 g
- Carbohydrates: 21.4 g

16. Blueberry Yogurt Mousse

Preparation Time: 4 minutes
Cooking Time: 0 minutes
Servings: 4
Ingredients:
- 2 cups Greek yogurt
- 1/4 cup stevia
- 3/4 cup heavy cream
- 2 cups blueberries

Directions:
1. In a blender, combine the yogurt with the other ingredients, pulse well, divide into cups, and keep it in the fridge for 30 minutes before serving.

Nutrition:
- Calories: 141
- Fat: 4.7 g
- Fiber: 4.7 g
- Carbs: 8.3 g
- Protein: 0.8 g

17. Stuffed Plums

Preparation Time: 4 minutes
Cooking Time: 20 minutes
Servings: 4
Ingredients:
- 4 plums, pitted, halved, not soft
- 1 tablespoon peanuts, chopped
- 1 tablespoon honey
- 1/2 teaspoon lemon juice
- 1 teaspoon coconut oil

Directions:
2. Make the packet from the foil and place the plum halves in it.
3. Then sprinkle the plums with honey, lemon juice, coconut oil, and peanuts.
4. Bake the plums for 20 minutes at 350°F.

Nutrition:
- Calories: 69
- Fat: 2.5 g
- Fiber: 1.1 g
- Carbs: 12.7 g
- Protein: 1.1 g

18. Cocoa Sweet Cherry Cream

Preparation Time: 4 minutes
Cooking Time: 0 minutes
Servings: 4
Ingredients:
- 1/2 cup cocoa powder
- 3/4 cup red cherry jam

- 1/4 cup stevia
- 2 cups water
- 1 pound cherries, pitted and halved

Directions:
1. Merge the cherries with the water and the rest of the ingredients, pulse well, divide into cups, and keep them in the fridge for 2 hours before serving.

Nutrition:
- Calories: 162
- Fat: 3.4 g
- Fiber: 2.4 g
- Carbs: 5 g
- Protein: 1 g

19. Mango and Honey Cream

Preparation Time: 4 minutes
Cooking Time: 30 minutes
Servings: 6
Ingredients:
- 2 cups coconut cream, chipped
- 6 teaspoons honey
- 2 mango, chopped

Directions:
1. Blend together honey and mango.
2. When the mixture is smooth, merge it with whipped cream and stir carefully.
3. Put the mango-cream mixture in the serving glasses and refrigerate for 30 minutes.

Nutrition:
- Calories: 272
- Fat: 19.5 g
- Fiber: 3.6 g
- Carbs: 27 g
- Protein: 2.8 g

20. Cinnamon Pears

Preparation Time: 4 minutes
Cooking Time: 25 minutes
Servings: 4
Ingredients:
- 2 pears
- 1 teaspoon ground cinnamon
- 1 tablespoon erythritol
- 1 teaspoon liquid stevia
- 4 teaspoons butter

Directions:
1. Cut the pears on the halves.
2. Then scoop the seeds from the pears with the help of the scooper.
3. In the shallow bowl mix up together erythritol and ground cinnamon.
4. Sprinkle every pear half with cinnamon mixture and drizzle with liquid stevia.
5. Then add butter and wrap in the foil.
6. Bake the pears for 25 minutes at 365°F.
7. Then remove the pears from the foil and transfer them to the serving plates.

Nutrition:
- Calories: 96
- Fat: 4 g
- Fiber: 3.6 g
- Carbs: 16.4 g
- Protein: 0.4 g

21. Classic Fig Clafoutis

Preparation Time: 4 minutes
Cooking Time: 45 minutes
Servings: 4
Ingredients:
- 2 large eggs
- 1/4 cup granulated sugar
- 2 tablespoons honey
- A pinch of grated nutmeg
- A pinch of flaky salt
- 1/3 cup all-purpose flour
- 1 tablespoon unsalted butter, at room temperature
- 1/4 cup whole milk
- 1/2 cup double cream
- 1/4 cup cognac
- 1 teaspoon orange zest, finely grated
- 8 figs, halved

Directions:
1. Preheat the oven.
2. In a mixing dish, thoroughly combine the eggs, sugar, honey, nutmeg, and salt.

3. Gradually stir in the flour and beat until creamy and smooth. Whisk in the butter, milk, double cream, cognac, and orange zest. Mix again to combine well.
4. Divide the batter into four lightly greased ramekins.
5. Top with the fresh figs and bake in the preheated oven for about 40 minutes until the clafoutis is golden at the edges. Bon appétit!

Nutrition:
- Calories: 328
- Fat: 10.4 g
- Carbs: 45.3 g
- Protein: 6.3 g

22. Semolina Cake with Almonds

Preparation Time: 30 minutes
Cooking Time: 2 hours 30 minutes
Servings: 4
Ingredients:
- 2 cups Greek yogurt
- 1 cup full-fat milk
- 1/2 cup coconut oil
- 1 1/2 cups powdered sugar
- 2 cups semolina
- 1 cup shredded coconut
- 1 teaspoon baking soda
- 1 teaspoon baking powder
- 1 tablespoon pure vanilla extract
- 1/4 teaspoon ground cinnamon
- 1/2 cup almonds, slivered

Directions:
1. Thoroughly combine the yogurt, milk, coconut oil, and sugar. Add in the semolina, shredded coconut, baking soda, baking powder, vanilla, and cinnamon.
2. Let it rest for 1 1/2 hour.
3. Bake until a tester inserted in the center of the cake comes out dry and clean.
4. Bring to a wire rack to cool completely before slicing and serving. Garnish with almonds and serve. Bon appétit!

Nutrition:
- Calories: 321
- Fat: 25 g
- Carbs: 46 g
- Protein: 6 g

23. Romantic Mug Cakes

Preparation Time: 30 minutes
Cooking Time: 5 minutes
Servings: 4
Ingredients:
- 2 eggs
- 1 1/2 tablespoons butter, melted
- 4 tablespoons full-fat milk
- 1 tablespoon rose water
- 1/4 teaspoon ground cinnamon
- 1/8 teaspoon grated nutmeg
- A pinch of coarse sea salt
- 4 tablespoons all-purpose flour

- 1/2 teaspoon baking powder
- 2 tablespoons cocoa powder
- 2 tablespoons powdered sugar
- 1 teaspoon grated orange zest

Directions:
1. Whisk the eggs, melted butter, milk, rose water, cinnamon, nutmeg, and salt.
2. Add in the flour, baking powder, cocoa powder, and sugar. Spoon the batter into two mugs.
3. Microwave for 1 minute 30 seconds and top with the grated orange zest. Bon appétit!

Nutrition:
- Calories: 264
- Fat: 14.4 g
- Carbs: 25.5 g
- Protein: 10.1 g

24. Pistachio and Tahini Halva

Preparation Time: 30 minutes
Cooking Time: 15 minutes
Servings: 6
Ingredients:
- 1/2 cup water
- 1/2 pound sugar
- 10 ounces tahini, at room temperature
- A pinch of sea salt
- 1/2 teaspoon vanilla paste
- 1/2 teaspoon crystal citric acid
- 1/3 cup shelled pistachios, chopped

Directions:
1. Place the water to a full boil in a small saucepan. Add in the sugar and stir. Let it cook, stirring occasionally, until a candy thermometer registers 250°F. Heat off.
2. Attach in the remaining ingredients and stir again to combine well. Now, scrape your halva into a parchment-lined square pan and smooth the top.
3. Let it cool with plastic wrap and place it in your refrigerator for at least 2 hours.

Nutrition:
- Calories: 464
- Fat: 28.4 g
- Carbs: 49.5 g
- Protein: 9.4 g

25. Authentic Greek Rizogalo

Preparation Time: 30 minutes
Cooking Time: 40 minutes
Servings: 3
Ingredients:
- 1 1/2 cups water
- 1/4 cup rice
- 2 cups whole milk
- 1/4 cup sugar
- A pinch of sea salt
- A pinch of grated nutmeg
- 1 egg, whisked
- 1 tablespoon butter

- 1/2 teaspoon vanilla extract
- 1/4 teaspoon ground cloves
- 1 teaspoon orange zest, grated
- 1/2 ground cinnamon

Directions:
1. Set the water and rice to a boil in a saucepan. Immediately turn the heat to a simmer. Let it simmer, stirring occasionally until most of the water has been absorbed, about 30 minutes.
2. Add in the milk, sugar, salt, and nutmeg, and bring to a boil again.
3. Add about 1 cup of the warm mixture to the beaten egg and whisk to combine well.
4. Lower the heat, add in the egg mixture, and continue simmering, stirring constantly, until the pudding has thickened.
5. Stir in the butter, vanilla, cloves, orange zest, and cinnamon, and serve at room temperature. Enjoy!

Nutrition:
- Calories: 247
- Fat: 10.4 g
- Carbs: 29.1 g
- Protein: 8 g

26.   Greek Frozen Yogurt Dessert

Preparation Time: 30 minutes
Cooking Time: 10 minutes
Servings: 3
Ingredients:
- 1/2 pineapple, diced
- 2 cups Greek-style yogurt, frozen

- 3 ounces almonds, slivered

Directions:
1. Divide the pineapple between two dessert bowls. Spoon the yogurt over it.
2. Top with the slivered almonds.
3. Cover and place in your refrigerator until you're ready to serve. Bon appétit!

Nutrition:
- Calories: 307
- Fat: 14.4 g
- Carbs: 29.1 g
- Protein: 18 g

27. Salted Pistachio and Tahini Truffles

Preparation Time: 30 minutes
Cooking Time: 30 minutes
Servings: 8
Ingredients:
- 1/2 cup pure agave syrup
- 1/2 cup dates, pitted and soaked
- 1/3 cup tahini
- 1/3 cup shelled pistachios, roasted and salted
- 1 teaspoon pure vanilla extract
- 1/2 teaspoon ground cinnamon
- A pinch of sea salt
- 2 tablespoons carob powder
- 2 tablespoons cocoa powder
- 2 cups rolled oats

Directions:
1. In your food processor, mix all of the above ingredients, except for the oats, until well combined.
2. Add in the rolled oats and stir with a wooden spoon.
3. Roll the mixture into small balls and place them your refrigerator until ready to serve. Bon appétit!

Nutrition:
- Calories: 224
- Fat: 9.5 g
- Carbs: 38.7 g
- Protein: 7.4 g

28. Traditional Olive Oil Cake with Figs

Preparation Time: 10 minutes
Cooking Time: 45 minutes
Servings: 9
Ingredients:
- 1/2 pound cooking apples, peeled, cored, and chopped
- 2 tablespoons fresh lemon juice
- 2 1/2 cups all-purpose flour
- 1 teaspoon baking powder
- 1/4 teaspoon sea salt
- 1/2 teaspoon ground cinnamon
- A pinch of grated nutmeg
- 3/4 cup granulated sugar
- 1/2 cup extra-virgin olive oil
- 2 eggs
- 1/2 cup dried figs, chopped
- 2 tablespoons walnuts, chopped

Directions:
1. Preheat the oven.
2. Then, thoroughly combine the flour, baking powder, sea salt, cinnamon, and nutmeg.
3. Then, beat the sugar and olive oil using your mixer at low speed.
4. Gradually fold in the eggs, one at a time, and continue to mix for a few minutes more until it has thickened.
5. Attach the wet mixture to the dry ingredients and stir until you get a thick batter. Fold in the figs and walnuts and stir to combine well.
6. Spoon the batter into a parchment-lined baking pan and level the top using a wooden spoon.
7. Bake until tester comes out dry and clean. Let it cool on a wire rack before slicing and serving. Bon appétit!

Nutrition:
- Calories: 339
- Fat: 15.6 g
- Carbs: 44.7 g
- Protein: 6.4 g

Chapter 3. Snacks

29.   Jazzed-Up Olives

Preparation Time: 5 minutes
Cooking Time: 10 minutes
Servings: 8
Ingredients:
- 1/2 cup extra-virgin olive oil
- 2 garlic cloves, minced
- 2 teaspoons fresh thyme leaves
- 1 teaspoon dried oregano
- 1/2 teaspoon red pepper flakes
- 2 cups mixed olives
- 1 tablespoon freshly squeezed lemon juice

Directions:
1. Heat the olive oil over low heat. Attach the garlic, thyme, oregano, and red pepper flakes and cook for about 2 minutes until the garlic starts to turn golden.
2. Add the olives and stir for about 1 minute to coat them in the oil mixture.
3. Transfer the olive mixture, including the oil, to a bowl and toss with the lemon juice.
4. Marinate for 1 hour before serving.

Nutrition:
- Calories: 160
- Total Fat: 17 g
- Protein: 0 g

30. Olive Tapenade

Preparation Time: 5 minutes
Cooking Time: 10 minutes
Servings: 2
Ingredients:
- 10 to 12 meaty olives, pitted and finely chopped
- 2 tablespoons extra-virgin olive oil
- 1 teaspoon freshly squeezed lemon juice
- 1 garlic clove, minced
- 1/2 teaspoon chopped capers
- 1/2 teaspoon anchovy paste
- 2 or 3 fresh basil leaves, chopped
- 1/2 teaspoon red pepper flakes
- Pinch freshly ground black pepper

Directions:
1. In a bowl, combine the olives, olive oil, lemon juice, garlic, capers, anchovy paste, basil, red pepper flakes, and black pepper and whisk well.

Nutrition:
- Calories: 144
- Total Fat: 16 g
- Protein: 1 g
- Carbohydrates: 1 g

31. Spicy Chickpeas

Preparation Time: 5 minutes
Cooking Time: 10 minutes

Servings: 6
Ingredients:
- 1 can chickpeas, rinsed and drained
- 3 tablespoons extra-virgin olive oil
- 1 teaspoon paprika
- 1/2 teaspoon salt
- 1/2 teaspoon cayenne pepper

Directions:
1. Set the chickpeas and detach as many of the soft skins as you can.
2. Heat the olive oil over low heat. Add the chickpeas and stir to coat. Slowly toast the chickpeas, stirring occasionally, until they get a little crunchy, about 10 minutes.
3. Use a spoon to transfer the chickpeas to a bowl lined with paper towels to absorb any excess oil.
4. Transfer the chickpeas to a serving bowl, sprinkle with the paprika, salt, and cayenne, and toss to coat.

Nutrition:
- Calories: 114
- Total Fat: 8 g
- Protein: 3 g
- Carbohydrates: 8 g

32. Layered Hummus Dip

Preparation Time: 5 minutes
Cooking Time: 10 minutes
Servings: 4
Ingredients:

- 1 cup classic hummus
- 1/2 cup finely chopped tomatoes
- 1/4 cup shredded Fontina cheese
- 2 tablespoons chopped pitted kalamata olives
- 1 tablespoon sweet hot cherry pepper relish

Directions:
1. Drizzle the hummus in the bottom of a small serving bowl.
2. Cover the hummus with the chopped tomatoes. Attach a layer of cheese, followed by a layer of kalamata olives.
3. Spoon the cherry pepper relish in the center. (Don't put the hot peppers all over the top, so guests can decide whether they want to add them.)

Nutrition:
- Calories: 144
- Total Fat: 8 g
- Protein: 5 g
- Carbohydrates: 14 g

33.   Kibbeh (Lebanese Croquettes)

Preparation Time: 1hour and 20 minutes
Cooking Time: 40 minutes
Servings: 4
Ingredients:
For the Kibbeh Dough:
- 1 1/2 cups fine bulgur
- 2 cups warm water
- 1 1/2 pounds ground beef
- 1 onion, cut into chunks
- 2 teaspoons ground allspice

- 1 teaspoon ground coriander
- 1 teaspoon freshly ground black pepper
- 1/2 teaspoon ground cinnamon
- Pinch salt

For the Stuffing:
- 2 tablespoons extra-virgin olive oil
- 1 onion, finely chopped
- 8 ounces ground beef or lamb
- 1/2 teaspoon ground allspice
- 1/4 teaspoon ground cinnamon
- Pinch salt
- Pinch freshly ground black pepper

Directions:
1. To make the dough: In a bowl, combine the bulgur and warm water and soak for 15 minutes. Drain. Wrap the bulgur in a kitchen towel and squeeze out the excess water.
2. In a food processor, combine the ground beef, onion, allspice, coriander, pepper, cinnamon, and salt. Process until the mixture forms a paste.
3. Mix by hand to form a dough. Cover and refrigerate while you make the stuffing.
4. Heat the olive oil over medium heat. Add the onion and cook for about 3 minutes, until it starts to soften. Add the ground meat and cook for 5 to 7 minutes until cooked through. Add the allspice, cinnamon, salt, and pepper and stir to combine. Detach from the heat and allow cooling.
5. Bring up an assembly line and the bowl of kibbeh dough, and the bowl of stuffing.

6. Dampen your hands with water. Shape 2 tablespoons of dough into a flat discups Wrap 1 tablespoon of stuffing inside the dough. Pinch to close.
7. Continue until you use all the ingredients, wetting your hands before forming each one. Place the kibbeh on the prepared baking sheet and refrigerate for 1 hour. Preheat the oven to 350°F.
8. Bake until golden brown.

Nutrition:
- Calories: 216
- Total Fat: 9 g
- Saturated Fat: 3 g
- Protein: 18 g
- Carbohydrates: 18 g

34. Cheese Plate with Fruit and Crackers

Preparation Time: 15 minutes
Cooking Time: 30 minutes
Servings: 8
Ingredients:
- 8 fresh figs, quartered
- 2 cups red and/or green grapes
- 8 ounces goat cheese
- 8 ounces Gorgonzola cheese
- 8 ounces Manchego cheese
- 8 ounces Parmigiano-Reggiano cheese
- 1 tablespoon Rosemary and thyme sprigs
- 1 cup pistachios
- 1 cup hazelnuts

- 1 cup almonds
- 2 cups red, green, and/or black olives
- 1 package whole wheat crackers
- 1 baguette, sliced

Directions:
1. Arrange the fruits and cheeses artfully on a wooden board. Scatter the herb sprigs here and there. Put the nuts and olives in small bowls and the crackers and baguette slices on a plate or in a basket.

Nutrition:
- Calories: 990
- Total Fat: 66 g
- Protein: 42 g
- Carbohydrates: 64 g

35. Radicchio Stuffed With Goat Cheese and Salmon

Preparation Time: 12 minutes
Cooking Time: 15 minutes
Servings: 8
Ingredients:
- 8 ounces goat cheese, at room temperature
- 2 tablespoons low-Fat: plain Greek yogurt
- 2 garlic cloves, peeled
- 1 tablespoon chopped fresh oregano
- 1 tablespoon chopped fresh basil
- 1 tablespoon chopped fresh rosemary
- 4 ounces smoked salmon

- 1 head radicchio, separated into leaves
- 1/4 teaspoon freshly ground black pepper

Directions:
1. Merge the goat cheese, yogurt, garlic, oregano, basil, and rosemary and blend until combined.
2. Set a piece of smoked salmon on each radicchio leaf. Top with 1 tablespoon of the cheese mixture. Sprinkle with black pepper.

Nutrition:
- Calories: 99
- Total Fat: 7 g
- Protein: 8 g
- Carbohydrates: 1 g

36. Rosemary–Sea Salt Crackers with Lemon-Parsley Dip

Preparation Time: 15 minutes
Cooking Time: 15 minutes
Servings: 4
Ingredients:
For the Dip:
- 8 ounces cream cheese
- 1/2 cup low-fat plain Greek yogurt
- 1/2 cup vegan mayonnaise
- 3 scallions, chopped
- 1/4 cup chopped fresh flat-leaf parsley
- 1 teaspoon chopped fresh thyme
- Finely grated zest of 1 lemon
- 1 teaspoon sea salt

- 1/4 teaspoon freshly ground black pepper

For the Crackers:
- 1 1/2 cups all-purpose flour
- 1 tablespoon finely chopped fresh rosemary
- 1 teaspoon coarse sea salt
- 1 teaspoon sugar
- 1/2 cup water
- 1 1/2 tablespoons extra-virgin olive oil

Directions:
1. Merge the cream cheese, yogurt, mayo, scallions, parsley, thyme, lemon zest, salt, and pepper and process until smooth.
2. Preheat the oven and in a rimmed baking sheet with parchment paper.
3. In a bowl, whisk together the flour, rosemary, salt, and sugar. Add the water and olive oil and stir to combine.
4. Turn out the dough onto a lightly floured work surface. Make out the dough until very thin, about 1/16 inches, adding more flour if the dough is too sticky.
5. Using a pizza cutter or no serrated knife, cut the dough into rectangles about 2 inches by 1 inch. Place on the prepared baking sheet. Brush with water and sprinkle with salt.
6. Bake until the crackers are golden.
7. Serve the crackers with the dip.

Nutrition:
- Calories: 535
- Total Fat: 35 g
- Protein: 12 g
- Carbohydrates: 43 g
- Fiber: 2 g

37. Spinach and Artichoke Dip

Preparation Time: 10 minutes
Cooking Time: 20 minutes
Servings: 8
Ingredients:

- Extra-virgin olive oil, for brushing
- 1 package frozen chopped spinach
- 1 jar marinated artichoke hearts
- 1 cup low-fat plain Greek yogurt
- 1 cup shredded fontina cheese
- 1/3 cup crumbled feta cheese
- 2 garlic cloves, minced
- Pinch salt
- 1/3 cup grated Parmesan cheese

Directions:

1. Preheat the oven to 350°F. Brush a 1-quart baking dish lightly with olive oil.
2. In a bowl, combine the spinach, artichoke hearts, yogurt, fontina, feta, garlic, and salt. Stir to combine thoroughly.
3. Pour into the prepared baking dish. Top with the Parmesan.
4. Bake until golden and bubbling.

Nutrition:

- Calories: 141
- Total Fat: 8 g
- Protein: 10 g
- Carbohydrates: 9 g
- Fiber: 4 g

38. Stuffed Cherry Tomatoes

Preparation Time: 15 minutes
Cooking Time: 15 minutes
Servings: 8
Ingredients:

- 24 cherry tomatoes
- 1/3 cup part-skim ricotta cheese
- 1/4 cup chopped peeled cucumber
- 1 tablespoon finely chopped red onion
- 2 teaspoons minced fresh basil

Directions:

1. Slice off the top of each tomato. Carefully scrape out and discard the pulp inside.
2. In a bowl, combine the ricotta, cucumber, red onion, and basil. Stir well.
3. Spoon the ricotta cheese mixture into the tomatoes and serve cold

Nutrition:

- Calories: 75
- Total Fat: 3 g
- Protein: 6 g
- Carbohydrates: 9 g
- Fiber: 1 g

39. Spiced Baked Pita Chips

Preparation Time: 10 minutes
Cooking Time: 10 minutes
Servings: 6

Ingredients:
- 2 tablespoons extra-virgin olive oil
- 1 teaspoon dried oregano
- 1/2 teaspoon paprika
- 1/2 teaspoon salt
- 1/4 teaspoon freshly ground black pepper
- 1/4 teaspoon cayenne pepper
- 3 pita breads, each cut into 8 triangles

Directions:
1. Preheat the oven to 350°F. Line a rimmed baking sheet with parchment paper.
2. Merge the olive oil, oregano, paprika, salt, black pepper, and cayenne. Mix well.
3. Spread out the pita triangles on the prepared baking sheet. Brush with the oil mixture. Flip over and brush the other side.
4. Bake until golden and crisp.

Nutrition:
- Calories: 78
- Total Fat: 5 g
- Protein: 1 g
- Carbohydrates: 8 g
- Fiber: 1 g

40. Roasted Red Pepper Dip

Preparation Time: 1 hour
Cooking Time: 45 minutes
Servings: 6

Ingredients:
- 4 large red bell peppers, seeded and quartered
- 1 large onion, chopped
- 2 tablespoons extra-virgin olive oil
- 1 teaspoon red wine vinegar
- 1 1/2 teaspoons salt
- 1/4 teaspoon freshly ground black pepper
- 2 garlic cloves, peeled

Directions:
1. Heat the oven and line a rimmed baking sheet with aluminum foil.
2. In a large bowl, toss the peppers and onion with olive oil, vinegar, salt, and pepper.
3. Spread out the peppers and onion in a single layer on the prepared baking sheet. Roast for 30 minutes, then add the garlic cloves and roast for another 15 minutes until the peppers start to blacken on the edges. Remove from the oven and set aside to cool.
4. Cool before serving.

Nutrition:
- Calories: 85
- Total Fat: 5 g
- Protein: 1 g
- Total Carbohydrates: 9 g
- Fiber: 3 g

41. Deviled Eggs with Spanish Smoked Paprika

Preparation Time: 15 minutes
Cooking Time: 15 minutes
Servings: 6
Ingredients:
- 6 large eggs
- 1 to 2 tablespoons mayonnaise
- 1 teaspoon Dijon mustard
- 1/2 teaspoon mustard powder
- 1/2 teaspoon salt
- 1/4 teaspoon freshly ground black pepper
- 1 teaspoon smoked paprika

Directions:
1. Cook the eggs and pour in enough water to completely submerge them.
2. When the eggs are processed, peel them and halve them lengthwise. Detach the yolks and put them in a small bowl.
3. To the yolks, add 1 tablespoon of mayonnaise, the Dijon mustard, mustard powder, salt, and pepper. Stir to blend completely, then add the remaining 1 tablespoon of mayonnaise if desired to achieve a smoother consistency. Spoon 1/2 tablespoon of the yolk mixture into each egg white.
4. Arrange the deviled eggs on a plate and sprinkle with the smoked paprika.

Nutrition:
- Calories: 89
- Total Fat: 7 g
- Protein: 6 g; Carbohydrates: 1 g

42.   Aperol Spritz

Preparation Time: 5 minutes
Cooking Time: 15 minutes
Servings: 4
Ingredients:
- Ice
- 3 ounces prosecco
- 2 ounces Aperol
- Splash club soda
- Orange wedge, for garnish

Directions:
1. Fill a wineglass with ice. Add the prosecco and aperol. Top with a splash of club soda. Garnish with an orange wedge.

Nutrition:
- Calories: 125
- Total Fat: 0 g
- Protein: 0 g
- Carbohydrates: 17 g
- Fiber: 0 g

43. VIN Brule

Preparation Time: 5 minutes
Cooking Time: 5 minutes
Servings: 4
Ingredients:
- 1 bottle dry red wine
- 3 cinnamon sticks
- 3 tablespoons sugar
- Peel of 1 orange

Directions:
1. Merge all the ingredients, cover, and boil.
2. Once it starts to boil, detach the lid, and carefully ignite with a flame. When the flame dies down, ladle into mugs.

Nutrition:
- Calories: 169
- Total Fat: 0 g
- Protein: 0 g
- Carbohydrates: 13 g
- Fiber: 0 g

44. Plum Wraps

Preparation Time: 5 minutes
Cooking Time: 10 minutes
Servings: 4
Ingredients:
- 4 plums
- 4 prosciutto slices
- 1/4 teaspoon olive oil

Directions:
1. Preheat the oven to 375°F.
2. Wrap every plum in prosciutto slices and secure with a toothpick (if needed).
3. Place the wrapped plums in the oven and bake for 10 minutes.

Nutrition:
- Calories: 62
- Fat: 2.2 g
- Fiber: 0.9 g
- Carbs: 8 g; Protein: 4.3 g

45. Easy Medi Kale

Preparation Time: 5 minutes
Cooking Time: 5 minutes
Servings: 2
Ingredients:

- 12 cups kale, chopped
- 2 tablespoons lemon juice
- 1 tablespoon olive oil
- 1 tablespoon garlic, minced
- 1 teaspoon soy sauce

Directions:

1. Add a steamer insert to your saucepan.
2. Pour water in the saucepan up to the bottom of the steamer.
3. Cover and bring water to boil (medium-high heat).
4. Add kale to the insert and steam for 7-8 minutes.
5. Take a large bowl and add lemon juice, garlic, olive oil, salt, soy sauce, and pepper.
6. Mix well and add the steamed kale to the bowl.
7. Toss and serve.

Nutrition:

- Calories: 32
- Fat: 8.2 g
- Fiber: 5.9 g
- Carbs: 18 g
- Protein: 9.3 g

46. Tropical Pineapple Smoothie

Preparation Time: 5 minutes
Cooking Time: 0 minutes

Servings: 1
Ingredients:
- 1 cup pineapple chunks, frozen
- 1/2 banana
- 1/4 cups mango chunks, frozen
- 1/2 cups orange juice
- 1/2 cups full-Fat: unsweetened coconut milk

Directions:
1. Combine the pineapple, banana, mango, orange juice, and coconut milk in a blender and process until smooth.
2. Pour into a glass and enjoy. Smoothies are best when you drink them right away.

Nutrition:
- Calories: 300
- Fat: 18 g
- Fiber: 2 g

47. Radish Bowls

Preparation Time: 5 minutes
Cooking Time: 3 minutes
Servings: 3
Ingredients:
- 1 cup radish
- 1 tablespoon fresh dill, chopped
- 1 teaspoon ground cinnamon
- 1 tablespoon butter

Directions:
1. Wash the radish carefully and slice it.
2. Toss the butter in the skillet and melt it.

3. Add sliced radish.
4. Sprinkle it with ground cinnamon and fresh dill. Mix up well.
5. Cook the radish for 3 minutes over medium heat.

Nutrition:
- Calories: 45
- Fat: 3.9 g
- Fiber: 1.2 g
- Carbs: 2.5 g
- Protein: 0.5 g

48. Cheddar Bites

Preparation Time: 5 minutes
Cooking Time: 15 minutes
Servings: 8
Ingredients:
- 3 phyllo sheets
- 1/2 cup cheddar cheese
- 2 eggs, beaten
- 1 tablespoon butter

Directions:
1. Mix up together cheddar cheese with eggs.
2. Spread the round springform pan with butter.
3. Place 2 phyllo sheets inside the springform pan.
4. Place the cheddar cheese mixture over the phyllo sheets and cover it with the remaining phyllo dough sheet.
5. Preheat the oven to 365°F.
6. Cut the phyllo dough pie onto 8 pieces and bake for 15 minutes.

Nutrition:
- Calories: 113
- Fat: 5.4 g
- Fiber: 0.4 g
- Carbs: 11.4 g
- Protein: 5 g

49. Creamy Pepper Spread

Preparation Time: 5 minutes
Cooking Time: 15 minutes
Servings: 4
Ingredients:
- 1 pound red bell peppers, chopped and remove seeds
- 1 1/2 tablespoons fresh basil
- 1 tablespoon olive oil
- 1 tablespoon fresh lime juice
- 1 teaspoon garlic, minced

Directions:
1. Situate all ingredients into the inner pot of the instant pot and stir well.
2. Seal the pot with the lid and cook on high for 15 minutes.
3. Once finished, let the pressure release naturally for 10 minutes, then release the rest using quick release. Remove the lid.
4. Transfer the bell pepper mixture into the food processor and process until smooth.
5. Serve and enjoy.

Nutrition:
- Calories: 41
- Fat: 3.6 g
- Carbohydrates: 3.5 g